Psychotherapy Under the Influence of Georges Bataille

This fascinating book applies social theorist Georges Bataille's revolutionary thinking to psychotherapy, offering clinicians a new and valuable context for practicing therapy.

In adding Bataille's ideas to several different psychotherapeutic modalities, this book makes the notoriously obscure thinker more accessible while testing the validity of his far-reaching work in the treatment room. Through an in-depth examination of several clinical case studies, the book demonstrates how to balance an understanding of the social and historical contexts of participants with a therapeutic approach that offers empathy for individual distress. It also explains how Bataille's innovative approach can be applied to work with couples, groups, institutions, and even one of Freud's classic case studies. Both the content and form of each chapter demonstrate the therapeutic value of a reflexive, critical approach to one's practice and exemplify how to write about it.

Offering an unprecedented opportunity to imagine how Bataille's own interest in psychoanalysis and clinical psychology might have developed, this book will be of interest to both practitioners in the field and scholars of continental philosophy and social theory.

William Buse, PhD, completed his anthropological training (Columbia University) and his psychoanalytic training (Postgraduate Center for Mental Health) in New York City. He currently serves as Director of Counseling at The Juilliard School and maintains a psychotherapy practice on the Upper West Side of Manhattan.

Psychotherapy Under the Influence of Georges Bataille

From Social Theory to Clinical Practice

William Buse

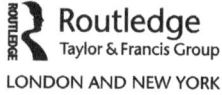

Routledge
Taylor & Francis Group

LONDON AND NEW YORK

First published 2021
by Routledge
2 Park Square, Milton Park, Abingdon, Oxon OX14 4RN

and by Routledge
52 Vanderbilt Avenue, New York, NY 10017

Routledge is an imprint of the Taylor & Francis Group, an informa business

© 2021 William Buse

British Library Cataloguing-in-Publication Data
A catalogue record for this book is available from the British Library

Library of Congress Cataloging-in-Publication Data
Names: Buse, William, 1955– author.
Title: Psychotherapy under the influence of
Georges Bataille: from social
theory to clinical practice / William Buse.
Description: Abingdon, Oxon; New York, NY: Routledge, 2021. |
Includes bibliographical references and index.
Identifiers: LCCN 2020045302 (print) |
LCCN 2020045303 (ebook) | ISBN 9780367740627 (hardback) |
ISBN 9780367347710 (paperback) | ISBN 9781003155942 (ebook)
Subjects: LCSH: Bataille, Georges, 1897–1962—Influence. |
Bataille, Georges, 1897–1962—Psychology. | Psychotherapy—
Methodology. | Psychology, Applied—Case studies.
Classification: LCC RC480.5 .B835 2021 (print) |
LCC RC480.5 (ebook) | DDC 616.89/14—dc23
LC record available at https://lccn.loc.gov/2020045302
LC ebook record available at https://lccn.loc.gov/2020045303

ISBN: 978-0-367-74062-7 (hbk)
ISBN: 978-0-367-34771-0 (pbk)
ISBN: 978-1-003-15594-2 (ebk)

Typeset in Times New Roman
by codeMantra

For my daughters

Contents

Figures

Acknowledgments

For their permission to re-publish the following articles, I wish to thank each of the following journals, who published an earlier form of these essays:

"Screened Out." In *European Journal of Psychoanalysis*. Online edition, September 2020.

"Sexual Disgust Redux." In *Psychoanalytic Review*, 481–507. Vol. 105 (5), October 2018.

"Searching for a Sign: Listening, Looking, Touching, Way-finding." In *Philosophy, Psychiatry & Psychology*, E-13–E-29. Vol. 25 (2), June 2018.

"The Distance between Spending and Spent: On Manic Consuming, Hoarding, Expending, and Other Visions of Excess." In *Philosophical Practice*, 1530–1538. Vol. 10 (1), March 2015.

"The Acephalic Stag." In *Group-Analysis*, 426–438. Vol. 46 (4), December, 2013.

First and foremost, I offer thanks to my patients, without whom there is quite literally nothing to write about; I owe them everything. My sincerest thanks to Mick Taussig at Columbia University for introducing me to the thought of Georges Bataille and, more importantly, for presenting a model of free thinking that changed the way I treat, teach, and write. Thank you Laurence Hegarty for patiently, critically, and constructively reading and providing feedback on most of the chapters herein. I am also grateful for the collaboration and support of the entire team I work with at the Counseling Service of The Juilliard School. Thanks to David Lynch for allowing me to use an image of Killer Bob to embellish my last chapter. Zoe Thomson and her editorial team at Routledge deserve special thanks for their thoughtful guidance shepherding this book to publication. And finally, most special thanks to my daughters Emily, Eleanor, and Evelyn for their constant loving support and belief in this project since its inception many years ago. They are all to be credited for any value this book may hold, while the faults I share alone.

O my brothers, am I cruel? But I say: what is falling, we should still push. Everything today falls and decays: who would check it? But I – I even want to push it. Do you know the voluptuous delight which rolls stones into steep depths? These human beings of today – look at them, how they roll into my depth! I am a prelude of better players, O my brothers! A precedent! Follow my precedent! And he whom you cannot teach to fly, teach to fall faster!

Friedrich Nietzsche, *Thus Spoke Zarathustra*, 1887

Introduction

This book was not originally intended as a manual for doing psychotherapy, and yet it has inadvertently become one. That is, it traces the cultivation of a unique psychotherapy hybrid that consists of one part psychoanalysis and one part applied anthropology. The result is a tentative, contingent, and exuberant perspective arrived at after years of conflating the activities of ethnography and psychotherapy in practice. I think this confusion of disciplines and their methods, theories, and arguments has been generative of predicaments and possibilities previously unconsidered and unrealized. And this, I believe, has been therapeutic; I leave it for you to decide.

This was also not intended to be a book about Georges Bataille. The man, the author by that name, remains as unknowable to me as he was for his mistress, Laure, who wrote to him, "I don't know if you don't understand anything or if you understand – too much" (Laure 1995, 148), and, likewise, one of his closest companions who posthumously grappled with the loss of his enigmatic friend:

> The 'I' whose presence his search seems still to make manifest when it expresses itself, toward whom does it direct us? Certainly toward an I very different from the ego that those who knew him in the happy and unhappy particularity of life would like to evoke in the light of a memory. Everything leads one to think that the personless presence at stake in such a movement introduces an enigmatic relation into the existence of him who indeed decided to speak of it but not to claim it as his own, still less to make of it an event of his biography.
>
> Blanchot (1997, 290–291)

I approached Bataille pragmatically, simply as one bricoleur to another. He consulted widely; from numerous artistic, religious, scholarly, and personal sources in order to understand the full range of human experience. His anguished life's search was expressed in his writing, whether that be pornography, surrealism, art and literary criticism, philosophy, or the social theory for which he has become most famous. After reading Bataille, I too felt I no longer would have to choose or declare myself within the constricted code of a single discipline or professional guild. His writing posed a model of boundless conceptualization about the human experience that I emulate in my clinical encounters every day. This, I believe, has enabled greater empathy with the elusive, often unknowable inner experience of my patients. Again, you will decide.'

In fact, there is a great deal of work I have left here for you, the reader. You are asked to enter and evaluate the following case studies depicting psychotherapy processes as an outsider, admitted only by way of their written representations. This is an impossible task insofar as the process of reading, while potentially therapeutic, is not parallel or even analogous with the process of being in therapy. Hence, what you will evaluate is not the therapy per se but simply how I have represented it – as its own categorically different semiotic practice. Perhaps this distinction is most directly indicative of the influence I attribute to Bataille. He, "'like Nietzsche, entrusted to his writing the essence of what he wanted to communicate'" (Jean Bruno quoted in Galletti 2018, 49). Accepting this shift in perspective, from therapy to writing, it could even seem then that the psychotherapy presented herein was conducted in the service of its written expression before you.

However, a third possibility exists, one that eludes an either/or dichotomy of perspectives. This comes to us from Bataille's own psychoanalytic treatment with Dr. Adrien Borel, in which both psychotherapy and writing were thoroughly conflated. A close look at this treatment provides an illustrative example of how both processes may inform one another.

To begin with, it seems that "several of Bataille's friends thought he was 'sick': he was a gambler, an alcoholic, and a frequenter of brothels ... he had even risked his life playing Russian roulette" (Roudinesco 1997, 121). Surely treatment seemed more necessary than elective.

Enter psychiatrist Adrien Borel who was a founding member of the Psychoanalytic Society of Paris. He was keenly interested in working with artists, and he took several members of the early Surrealist movement into treatment with him:

> what led him to greet the advent of the movement favorably was the study of dreamers rather than of dreams per se ... he wrote 'We have just learned of a new movement: Surrealism, as explained and commented on by its creator, Andre Breton ... we feel obliged to take note of the escape from the real the author has attempted in order to enclose himself (or rather expand himself) into an extremely extended imaginary universe toward whose elaboration every means of expression and all that is marvelous or enchanted in the individual join to contribute.'
>
> Roudinesco (1990, 8–9)

Bataille (1986), writing of himself in the third person, provides this general statement about his treatment in an "Autobiographical Note":

> The virulently obsessive character of his writing troubles one of his friends, Dr. Dausse, who has him undergo psychoanalysis with Dr. Borel. The psychoanalysis has a decisive result; by August 1927 it put an end to the series of dreary mishaps and failures in which he had been floundering, but not to the state of intellectual intensity, which still persists.
>
> (108)

Borel's exceptional interest in the shared unconscious zone constituted by dreaming, culture, and artistic expression informed a perspective free from conventional psychoanalytic parameters. This may explain his active but non-intrusive participation in Bataille's writing process that became de facto the treatment. Bataille (1998) states,

> I undertook psychoanalysis, which was perhaps not very orthodox, because it lasted only a year. It was a little short, but in the end it changed me from being as absolutely obsessive as I was into someone relatively viable. It profoundly moved me and completely released me ... the first book I wrote ... I was able to write it only when psychoanalyzed, yes, as I came out of it. And I believe I am able to say that it is only by being liberated in this way that I was able to write.
>
> (221)

"Borel encouraged Bataille to write, without trying to end the state of intellectual violence from which he claimed to be suffering ... the text [Story of the Eye] was discussed at every session – and sometimes revised too" (Roudinesco 1997, 122). In Borel, it would seem that Bataille found a caring, kindred spirit:

> [Borel] was especially a heterodox Freudian: he relished dogma as little as Bataille, even that of the founder ... With him, treatment was above all else 'therapeutic, adaptive and founded with attention to suffering.' It was, in short, 'not very rigorous' and not 'ritualized,' *a fortiori* with creative people ... who he allowed to struggle with the unconscious ... The analysis could therefore roughly have been this: on Borel's side, an encouragement to write; on Bataille's, a writing producing a series of images in response, which in turn oiled the keys of the analysis, keys which probably threw a new light on the book, enabling him to carry it to a conclusion. To some extent it was, if the word could be used, an 'applied' analysis ... Borel assumed an attentive and kindly position.

He encouraged and commented: he steadied and supported the heavy obsessional material of the narrative (which could well have alarmed him) when necessary. Everything did not immediately fall into place. He sometimes contributed to the findings ... Adrien Borel, reacting to the writing, encouraged admission, and, when necessary, worked on all the possible meanings with Bataille.

Surya (2002, 97–98, including citation of Roudinesco 1986)

What Surya characterizes as an 'applied' analysis seemed to be an innovation of this treatment that would have resonance throughout Bataille's writing career. According to Kendall (2007), Bataille's,

knowledge of psychoanalysis prior to undergoing treatment was literally introductory and Dr. Borel might be understood as the intermediary who initiated Bataille in his study of this approach to anthropological analysis ... His interest in psychoanalysis would be as a means of cultural or anthropological analysis rather than one of personal analysis.

(51)

Many years after the treatment concluded, Bataille would join with Borel and others to form the Society of Collective Psychology. Their mission, according to Bataille, was "to study the role of psychological factors, and particularly unconscious ones, in social facts; to converge research heretofore undertaken in isolation in diverse disciplines" (Bataille quoted in Dean 1994, 216). The Society was short-lived, perhaps meeting only once, but long enough to set a theme for their research: "Attitudes when faced with death" (Hollier 1988, 103–104).

The scholarly, artistic, and personal exploration of human attitudes when faced with death would preoccupy Bataille for the rest of his life. However, this preoccupation was derivative of a theme that surfaced in his treatment with Dr. Borel as early as 1927. The following dream associations emerged during Bataille's treatment at that time:

Terrors of childhood spiders, etc. linked to the memory of having my pants down on my father's knees.

Kind of ambivalence between the most horrible and the most magnificent.

I'm something like three years old my legs naked on my father's knees and my penis bloody like the sun. This for playing with a hoop. My father slaps me and I see the sun.

Bataille (1991, 4)

Based on verbal and written comments like those above, Borel would surely have been aware of the strong potential for a paternal transference to develop in his treatment of Bataille. It is therefore remarkable that, whether acting consciously or unconsciously, either in a gesture of great empathy or from countertransference, Borel presented Bataille with a gift during the treatment – a photographic image of a Chinese man undergoing *Lingchi*, known in English as the "death by a thousand cuts." This was to have a profound and lasting impact:

> The world evoked by this straightforward image of a tortured man, photographed several times during the torture, in Peking, is, to my knowledge, the most anguishing of worlds accessible to us through images captured on film … Since 1925, I have owned one of these many pictures. It was given to me by Dr. Borel, one of the first French psychoanalysts. The photograph had a decisive role in my life. I have never stopped being obsessed by this image of pain, at once ecstatic (?) and intolerable … Much later, in 1938, a friend initiated me into the practice of yoga. It was on this occasion that I discerned, in the violence of this image, an infinite capacity for reversal. Through this violence – even today I cannot imagine a more insane, more shocking form – I was so stunned that I reached the point of ecstasy … What I suddenly saw, and what imprisoned me in anguish – but which at the same time delivered me from it – was the identity of these perfect contraries, divine ecstasy and its opposite, extreme horror.
>
> Bataille (1992, 205–207)

This finally brings us back to the task before you, the reader. To identify here with the patient, Bataille, is to accept that in *his* identification with a man tortured beyond all anguish to the point of ecstasy, he felt affirmed or, in his own words, "released." After all, he kept the photo on his writing desk in front of him and featured it prominently in the last publication of his life (1992). Through the image, and particularly the personal associations to the image as worked out with his therapist Borel, Bataille found it possible to articulate his experience. It would be enough to stop at this understanding and be grateful for his good fortune receiving this gift through which the poor fate of the tortured man was redeemed. But there's more.

It is impossible for me to overlook the multidetermined motivation behind this special gift from Borel to Bataille. Hence, to identify with Borel is to accept that, whether consciously or unconsciously, a gift given in treatment, as with a dream, must be considered a representation of the treatment itself. Regarding the photo as such, depth interpretation thereby becomes synonymous with laceration, insight with euphoric release from anguish: "my father slaps me and I see the sun." Borel sensed that Bataille's personal anguish was not to be pathologized or avoided but, counterintuitively, to be entered, and that this entry and his patient's subsequent release would be enabled by the strange depiction of joint anguish and ecstasy in the photograph. As if to underscore the profound generative significance of Borel's gift, Bataille reciprocated by writing prolifically thereafter, with the photograph directly in front of him, and then sending the first copy of every book he published to Borel.

My wish is that the anguish and suffering experienced and shared by the people I have been fortunate to treat may ultimately be generative, not only of insight and agency for them, or of the cathartic expression provided for me in writing this book, but of an unforeseen and exuberant release for you, the reader.

* * *

In the spirit of the "applied analysis" undertaken in this book, it is organized into different parts based on the modalities of treatment I adopted. Each modality represents an opportunity to explore and redefine what is considered therapeutic with respect to the individual *and* social aspects of the encounter. Throughout, Borel (as I imagine him) provided a model for my style of engagement, while Bataille provided a conceptual language for describing and interpreting it. Individual psychotherapy is the first and most frequently used modality in my work. Thus, Part 1 consists of the bulk of case studies. The other modalities – couples, group, and community psychotherapy – are all represented by the following individual chapters in separate parts. The final part of the book, on the end(s) of psychotherapy, attempts to explore the purpose of a treatment through an examination of how it is ended. To this end, I juxtapose a contemporary case study with the famous account of the first patient to undergo a psychoanalytic treatment, Anna O.

Bibliography

Bataille, Georges. "Autobiographical Note." In *October*, 107–110. Edited by Annette Michelson. Vol. 36, Spring, 1986.

Bataille, Georges. "Dream." In *Visions of Excess: Selected Writings, 1927–1939*, 3–4. Edited and translated by Allan Stoekl. Minneapolis, MN: University of Minnesota Press, 1991/1927.

Bataille, Georges. *The Tears of Eros*. Translated by Peter Connor. San Francisco, CA: City Lights Books, 1992/1961.

Bataille, Georges. "Interview with Madeleine Chapsal." In *Georges Bataille: Essential Writings*, 220–224. Edited by Michael R. Richardson. Thousand Oaks, CA: Sage Publications, 1998/1961.

Blanchot, Maurice. *Friendship.* Translated by Elizabeth Rottenberg. Stanford, CA: Stanford University Press, 1997/1971.

Dean, Carolyn J. *The Self and Its Pleasures: Bataille, Lacan, and the History of the Decentered Subject.* Ithaca, NY: Cornell University Press, 1994.

Galletti, Marina. "The Secret Society of Acephale: 'A Community of the Heart'." In *The Sacred Conspiracy: The Internal Papers of the Secret Society of Acephale and Lectures to the College of Sociology*, 19–49. Edited by Marina Galletti and Alastair Brotchie. Translated by John Harman. London: Atlas Press, 2018.

Hollier, Denis. "Preface to Attraction and Repulsion I: Tropisms, Sexuality, Laughter and Tears." In *The College of Sociology, 1937–1939*, 103–104. Edited by Denis Hollier. Translated by Betsy Wing. Minneapolis, MN: University of Minnesota Press, 1988.

Kendall, Stuart. *Georges Bataille*. London: Reaktion Books, 2007.

Laure. "Letter to Georges Bataille." In *Laure: The Collected Writings*, 147–149. Edited by Jerome Peignot. Translated by Jeanine Herman. San Francisco, CA: City Lights Books, 1995/1934.

Roudinesco, Elisabeth. *La Bataille de Cent Ans. Histoire de la Psychoanalyze en France*. Paris: Seuil. 1986 (French).

Roudinesco, Elisabeth. *Jacques Lacan & Co.: A History of Psychoanalysis in France, 1925–1985*. Translated by Jeffrey Mehlman. Chicago, IL: The University of Chicago Press, 1990.

Roudinesco, Elisabeth. *Jacques Lacan*. Translated by Barbara Bray. New York: Columbia University Press, 1997.

Surya, Michael. *Georges Bataille: An Intellectual Biography*. Translated by Krzysztof Fijalkowski and Michael Richardson. New York: Verso, 2002.

Part I

Psychotherapy with individuals

Chapter 1

Searching for a sign

Listening, looking, touching, way-finding

This is an account of the psychotherapeutic treatment of a sign-maker. The treatment posed a special challenge due to the patient's idiosyncratic blend of sexual, artistic, and spiritual interests, all of which informed his own notion of the sign/way-finding relationship. Way-finding came to connote more than its usual pedestrian meaning—it came to represent a spiritual quest and a personal exploration of the sacred. Conceptualizing this treatment, first for myself (the clinician), then for the patient, and now for you the reader, led me through a way-finding process of my own. This entailed a reconsideration of the function and meaning of signs before finally locating the pertinent theoretical context for my understanding of the patient. Ultimately, it was in the work of French social theorist Georges Bataille, particularly in his 1930 essay "Base Materialism and Gnosticism," that I was able to acquire the conceptual framework that properly expressed the sacred as understood by my patient and that informed all aspects of his life, including his treatment. However, first and foremost, the patient was a sign-maker, and so it is with the conventional interpretation and function of signs, and the way-finding they enable, that I begin.

In 1960, Kevin Lynch published his ground-breaking book entitled *The Image of the City*. For this study of urban design he coined an unusual term: "way-finding." Way-finding captures the conceptual novelty of Lynch's discussion; that is, he writes of the city as a landscape to be traversed both physically and in a simultaneously parallel, Kantian way, within one's mind: "In the process of way-finding, the strategic link is the environmental image, the generalized mental picture of the physical world that is held by the individual" (1960, 5). This internal image of the city is "read" by the way-finder to the extent that it is, as Lynch proposes, "legible."

Legibility, and the clarity and ease of comprehension it enables, is in turn facilitated by the invention or discovery of signs that are positioned throughout our environment. A sign is "an object, quality, or event whose presence or occurrence indicates the probable presence or occurrence of something else" (Oxford English Dictionaries online). For the way-finder, according to Lynch, this could consist of a path, an edge, a node, or a boundary. However, following Lynch, if we additionally consider the interior landscape of the way-finder, our experience of signs might also include dreams, symptoms, memories, fears, or wishes (on the subjective contribution to sign interpretation from the field of linguistics see theorists Saussure 1915 and Peirce 1897; the latter especially regarding his "trichotomous interpretation of signs").

Beyond the information from exterior and interior frames of individual experience lies the world of the supernatural as articulated by myth. This suggests a third mode of way-finding that expands the notion to include such activities as a pilgrimage, a mission, or a quest. This conventionally recognized spiritual dimension is exemplified by Chatwin's (1987) discussion of Australian Aboriginal "songlines," or paths through a landscape that are simultaneously past and present, natural and supernatural, and navigated by simultaneous actions of precise ritual singing and walking. As suggested by Chatwin, supernatural phenomena such as the aboriginal mythic Dreamtime stretch the way-finder's sojourn beyond real time, with the sign serving both as an omen auguring future tidings as well as an enduring if not arcane signature of the ancestors from the past. Aboriginal way-finding is thus the equivalent of worship – an acknowledgement of one's origins in Dreamtime – as well as an affirmation of the relational order by which the aborigine is oriented (kinship relations include animistic aspects of the flora and fauna of the aboriginal environment).

Notwithstanding this plasticity of the sign – whether appearing in a city landscape, a Freudian dream, or aboriginal Dreamtime – it is generally construed as functionally generative of symbolic meaning and thereby orders our world. This ubiquity of symbolic function, implying as it does "the probable presence or occurrence of something else," as well as its ordering, synthesizing function, are common qualities that account for the homogeneity of all human signs. So effective, so pervasive are these features that our understanding of ourselves and our world is thoroughly shaped by that which pragmatically fulfills a signifying and synthesizing function; that is, until we encounter an event or object that exceeds or subverts this universal function of the sign. That place where our signs cease to orient and affirm lies in the realm of the sacred.

Perhaps because of its seemingly anomalous social character, cultural anthropologists in particular have approached the sacred with special interest. Geertz (1989, 10) refers to "the peculiar 'otherness,' the extraordinary, momentous, 'set apart' quality of sacred acts and objects." Even more pointedly, fellow anthropologist Douglas (1966, 48) famously postulated the criteria for a universal definition of the sacred as being "matter out of place." I wish to focus presently on only two aspects of this latter definition; that is, the suggestion of disorder and the emphasis on matter. Taken together, these heterogeneous features of the sacred dialectically threaten, necessitate, and ultimately shape the homogeneous world of signs and the activity of way-finding, for, as Douglas (1966) states (equating notions of the sacred with notions of dirt),

> Dirt [the sacred], then, is never a unique isolated event. Where there is dirt [the sacred] there is a system. Dirt [the sacred] is the by-product of a systematic ordering and classification of matter [signs], in so far as ordering involves rejecting inappropriate elements.
>
> 48

Exploring the relationship of these features of the sacred and their subversive potential was the preoccupation of French social theorist Georges Bataille. By way of an introduction, Bataille eludes easy categorization. During his most active period stretching from the late 1920s through the World War II, he was a formative part of Andre Breton's surrealist movement, published pornographic texts under a pseudonym, earned a living as a medieval librarian, founded both highly influential journals, *Documents* and *Critique*, and founded the secret society *Acephale*, a workshop of sorts through which he sought to enact his ideas. He is best known for both the content and form of his essays on social theory that embody a highly original integration of varied and diverse European intellectual strands including the works of Freud, Marx, Nietzsche, Hegel, and Sade, along with contributions from numerous ethnographic, theological, and literary sources. Moreover, Bataille's focus was on a specific aspect of the European intellectual stream. It was Hegel's work on the negative, Nietzsche's exploration of nihilism, as well as Freud's notion of the death instinct that seemed to have most affected him. His work has been acknowledged as a prominent influence by later French intellectuals Barthes, Lacan, Foucault, and Derrida among others and, in part due to the highly idiosyncratic form and critical focus of his work, has often been dubbed the precursor to post-structuralism.

While certainly never intended for use in the clinic, this author has found Bataille's ideas very helpful as a non-reductive means of understanding and empathizing with individuals experiencing psychological states very different from his own. Specifically, Bataille sought to reinstate the central importance of expenditure (*depense*), waste, excess, and base materialism; all, he argued, once among the core components of a "general economy" in pre-modern human life. In so doing, he was offering a critical, remedial response to the limited focus based on scarcity and accumulation that is associated with the "restricted economy" of global capitalism.

In our contemporary world, production and subsistence are the *sine qua non* activities by which all other human endeavors are measured. Bataille contested this view as partial, incomplete, and ultimately dehumanizing. Pointing to numerous case studies ranging from ancient history to current annals of criminal and deviant behavior, he sought to theorize those ubiquitous and enduring human activities that cannot be rationalized as productive and offer no functional or utilitarian value, such as sacrifice, festival, eroticism, war, and self-mutilation. His project may be seen as having far-reaching implications for psychology to the extent that, post-Enlightenment, all the positivist sciences fall under the pervasive influence of the ethos characterizing a restricted economy. Hence, an unrestricted psychology would rightly be concerned with the micro elements of human experience and behavior that are stigmatized and suppressed within the macro value structure associated with the restricted economy of contemporary society.

In the following case example, the patient developed his own novel and highly personal notion of the sacred that was simultaneously spiritual, sexual, and aesthetically determined, and even materially actualized in his everyday life. This required an inquiring, supportive response unfettered by the limits of this clinician's own values. I aspired to an open, receptive stance by consulting Bataille's work, beginning with the writings and discussions of the College of Sociology, an intellectual discussion group Bataille founded that met from 1937 to 1939 in Paris and whose participants included Claude Lévi-Strauss, Alexandre Kojeve, and Walter Benjamin, among others (see Hollier 1988). A central mission of the College was the development of a "Sacred Sociology, implying the study of all manifestations of social existence where the active presence of the sacred is clear" (1988a, 5). Reformulating the sacred as inherently exuding the threat of disorder, Bataille (1988b, 122) stated, "the integrity of human existence is put at stake each time sacred things are originally produced." Bataille's described this sacred disorder as "heterogeneous" and defined it in relation to the "homogeneity" of social order:

> In summary, compared to everyday life, *heterogeneous* existence can be represented as something *other*, as *incommensurate* ... a *force* that disrupts the regular course of things ... The very term *heterogeneous* indicates that it concerns elements that are impossible to assimilate ... the heterogeneous world is largely comprised of the sacred world ... Beyond the properly sacred things that constitute the common realm of religion and magic, the *heterogeneous* world includes everything resulting from *unproductive* expenditure. This consists of everything rejected by *homogeneous* society as waste ... Included are the waste products of the human body and certain analogous matter (trash, vermin, etc.); the parts of the body; persons, words, or acts having an erotic value; [as well as] the violent and excessive nature of a decomposing body ... The reality of *heterogeneous* elements is not of the same order as that of *homogeneous* elements. *Homogeneous* reality presents itself with the abstract and neutral aspect of strictly defined and identified objects. *Heterogeneous* reality is that of a force or shock. It presents itself as a charge, as a value.
>
> 1991b (140–143, author's emphases)

Bataille's (1991a) reformulation of the sacred with regard to materiality is specifically developed toward the goal of re-assimilating, or at least recognizing as significant, the censored, discarded, deviant, excessive, or wasteful aspects of modern life and hence his discussion of the affinity between what he terms "base materialism" and Gnosticism. This is not a dead materialism on which is built a hierarchy, decidedly Christian, which relies on a disparagement of all that is profane and culminates in the lofty equation of consciousness with an elite realization of the sacred through enlightenment. As with Douglas's (1966) aforementioned characterization of the sacred as matter out of place, Bataille also equates the sacred with dirt or, in his words "base matter," and emphasizes the importance of the dialectical relationship between heterogeneous disorder and homogeneous order:

> Base matter is external and foreign to ideal human aspirations, and it refuses to allow itself to be reduced to the great ontological machines resulting from these aspirations. But the psychological process brought to light by Gnosticism had the same impact: it was a question of disconcerting the human spirit and idealism before something base, to the extent that one recognized the helplessness of superior principles.
>
> 1991a (51)

Examples of Gnostic base matter that are invoked by Bataille include "obscene and lawless archontes ... the head of the solar ass (whose comic and desperate braying would be the signal for a shameless revolt against idealism in power) ... certain sexual rites ... black magic" (48) and relic stones surviving from the third and fourth centuries, most likely of Egyptian origin, that depict an acephalic god (48–52).

For Bataille, "it is possible to see as a *leitmotiv* of Gnosticism the conception of matter as an *active* principle having its own eternal autonomous existence" (47, author's emphasis). Historically, this understanding of matter, or base matter of the Gnostics, was dangerously subversive and "compromised newborn Christian theology and Hellenistic metaphysics" (46). By invoking the base materiality of the Gnostics to redefine the sacred, and thereby attempting to reinstate all of its creative and subversive potential, Bataille provided us with conceptual recourse from the same dominant idealist Christian values that initially supplanted Gnosticism in antiquity; idealist values that have steadily flourished post-Enlightenment into what Weber (1918) identified as the "disenchantment of the world."

This author (as clinician) operated on the hypothesis that this subversive potential of base matter, as experienced in everyday life, was not only relevant for the Gnostics but held therapeutic potential in the treatment situation. Following Bataille, the notion of base matter was invoked as a remedial heuristic construct within a society or, microscopically, an individual life that had become morally constipated for lack of an opportunity to expend itself in a non-productive manner, or, in other words, a life solely devoted to production and bereft of any encounter with the sacred.

According to this clinical appropriation of Bataille's thought, the risk of psychopathology advances with each step further into the modern homogeneous world based solely on production, especially production ideologically rationalized and reinforced through the processes of abstraction, metaphor, and symbolism; with the seeker/way-finder accordingly becoming increasingly alienated from direct experience of the heterogeneous sacred in everyday life. Today it is as though any experience of the sacred must necessarily be mediated; in fact, the mediating sign itself has become fetishized and mistaken for the sacred (see McLuhan 2002 and Baudrillard 1995 regarding examples and ramifications of this historical and cultural development; and particularly Benjamin 2002 for his discussion on the "aura" of original artwork versus the mechanically reproduced image). Yet without the heterogeneous "charge" of the sacred experience, without any contact with "matter out of place," the sign becomes nothing more than a floating signifier that can only "represent an indeterminate value of signification, in itself devoid of meaning and thus susceptible of receiving any meaning at all" (Lévi-Strauss 1987, 55). The sign is now revealed as unstable and arbitrary (hence Saussure's famous pronouncement: "The linguistic sign is arbitrary" (1966, 67). It is only as our signs, or our faith in signs begins to fail that we will gradually understand the extent to which our deification of the sign now permeates the physical, psychological, and supernatural life of we modern human way-finders; that is, the realization of the depth of our total dependency on arbitrary and unstable signs for a homogeneous sense of basic orientation in time and space, personal meaning, even our sense of identity as a species, will ironically result in the collective experience of being lost.

When Ward contacted me, he was lost. He could or would not even tell me why he wanted to consult me. And so I embarked, as all psychotherapists do, on my own professionally sanctioned, idiosyncratic version of way-finding; I began to construct Ward through the composite of symptoms that he consciously and unconsciously presented – my assessment process itself reflecting the earliest form of sign-reading (see Barthes 1964 and Sebeok 1994 on the foundational importance of symptom-reading for a science of semiotics). Gradually I pieced together bits and pieces of identifying data that together formed an initial, tentative profile. I learned that Ward was a 51-year-old gay man who lived alone though he had a partner, a man many years his senior that he had seen regularly for several years. In our first meeting and always thereafter, Ward was fashionably attired, eloquent, and deliberate in his movements – the picture of urbane elegance. As a young man, he acquired fluency in Italian after certificate training in design in Italy, and approached fluency in Spanish after two years in Panama for the Peace Corps. His mother called him Eddy, his friends and colleagues addressed him as Ed, but in our relationship, he wanted to be known as Ward. Utilizing the second half of Edward enabled Ward to retain a continuous sense of himself but with a different accent. "Ward" was closer to the internal ideal of the man that he aspired to be and, hopefully with my help, would fully realize. This, it would seem, was why Ward, Ed, and Eddy had decided to contact me.

Ward lived alone on a quiet shady block in Brooklyn Heights in a very small, thoughtfully decorated studio apartment shared only with his books and meticulously maintained fish tank. He had few friends, was exceedingly private, preferred silence, had no television, and never answered his telephone at home.

His social isolation notwithstanding, Ward's greatest sources of human interaction were through his two passions: art and theology. His love of art led to a BFA in environmental design in New York; his love of theology led to an intense study of comparative religion in a Roman Catholic seminary that, although aborted, would be a central preoccupation for the rest of his life.

By the time we met, Ward had worked for decades as an environmental graphic designer. He was a self-identified maker of signs. Under the auspices of the small private company that employed him in Manhattan, he produced signs for schools, hospitals, banks, office buildings, parks, and so on. However, after years of making signs, Ward had grown weary and resentful of the criticisms, concessions, and compromises to his artistic vision that he continually and patiently endured. Especially demoralizing was the recent mandate to comply with an enormously elaborate and intricate set of bureaucratic requirements and regulations that governed all signage for accessibility as mandated by the American Disabilities Act (ADA-Architectural Barriers Act 2004). Employment anomie, coupled with his partner's increasingly debilitating Parkinson's Disease, gradually led Ward to smoke and drink heavily on a daily basis.

Ostensibly, it seemed that Ward's smoking, drinking, and social isolation were the dominant signs of distress or, clinically framed, presenting symptoms of a major depression. However, the most alarming behaviors at first glance often signify the patient's best effort at a solution to a much deeper, more insidious, invisible dilemma. In Ward's case, that deeper dilemma was his increasing lack of conviction in the meaning and/or relevance of his labor, if not his life.

And his spending his health, in what could only appear as a vain, futile effort, brought no relief. For Ward, all signs now only signified more signs, an endless forest of signs never arriving at significance. I diagnosed this existential lack of conviction as a severe form of pathologically obsessive semiosis, characterized by an excessive focus on signifiers to the detriment of significance and meaning. Feeling increasingly dissociated, Ward examined life ironically as a poorly executed aesthetic production and often responded with a scathing critical review, especially regarding himself as the featured grade B actor of this second-rate production.

My efforts to connect with any positive, non-ironic emotional attachments that Ward valued usually failed. His response when asked why he went to the gym every day: "I want to be the best-looking corpse at the funeral home." On his occasional forays out of the city with his partner: "nature is over-rated." On his sexual experiment with weekly visits to an older female prostitute across town: "I go to see how she wears her hair, her choice of clothing, and her make-up." On his religious beliefs: "Because of my interest in various religious traditions, it is fair to say, my opinions are more catholic than Catholic," adding, "Although not necessarily a personal objective; I find martyrdom admirable." Moreover, Ward often dismissed therapy or more exactly, my efforts at intervening therapeutically, as irrelevant but enjoyed the ritualized theatricality that informed my style of conducting the treatment – especially in that I seemed to take it seriously.

As auxiliary ego for Ward, I set out to establish the treatment relationship as a laboratory within which he could feel or care again and, by way of Bataille's influence, a place in which his expending himself mattered.

The one area of his life that was not qualified was that which Ward referred to as his spiritual journey or search. As his partner's condition deteriorated and finally culminated in death, Ward returned to the Catholic Church and his long-standing spiritual interests. Turned off by what he referred to as "the excessive mythology" of the modern mass, he struggled to stay involved in his local parish. However, our sessions often ended up being devoted to a review of the poor lighting or unruly congregation that ruined the experience. When finally a Good Friday mass service improvised a modern ritual in which members of the congregation were invited to approach the altar and kiss the cross held by the priest, he withdrew from the church on grounds that it had resorted to kitsch – tacky and unconvincing theater. As a parody of this event, he kept a chocolate crucifix in his freezer for years which he ceremoniously took out and licked on Good Friday.

Ward's dissatisfaction with the Church led him to other forums through which he could continue to satisfy his spiritual proclivity. He attended dharma discussions at a local ashram and, while he never participated, he was engaged and amused by the open discussion. This was indeed social interaction, if inconsequential and at a distance. Eventually he left the dharma experience claiming he couldn't get into the blue elephants gracing the iconic portraits on the walls. However, Ward had now identified a focus that he could objectively and non-ironically embrace: he was on a non-denominational spiritual journey, however unconventional and idiosyncratic that might appear. I was employed as witness to his journey and my interest was initially and provisionally accepted (and expected) as an auxiliary surrogate for his own missing or tentative conviction (or faith).

Ward quit drinking and smoking, and began attending regular yoga and meditation classes. At some point, he began developing his own meditation practice at home. As his self-styled spiritual practice developed, he visited Italy several times, making pilgrimages to monasteries, churches, and historical sites such as Pompeii. This is not to suggest that Ward had been suddenly and completely transformed. He still focused on the Vatican gift shop during each visit to Rome to see if he could get the same magenta-colored socks worn by the Pope – the greatest arbiter of fashion in Ward's estimation. Moreover, Ward declared that his "fantasies of developing a 'way-finding' program for the Vatican would be a theological challenge." It soon became apparent that what Ward referred to as his 'spiritual development' included a higher, more refined involvement with the aesthetic, material trappings or props of conventional worship.

This period included Ward's delving into Christianity by way of art history, philosophy, and historical novels which sexualized popularly esteemed sacred figures. Of particular interest to Ward was Leo Steinberg's (1997) discussion of the phallus of Christ. This work, perhaps more than any other, forged a path for Ward back into the Church. To the extent that his homosexuality, or rather sexuality in general, was prohibited during his early experience as a Roman Catholic, Ward had always felt like a failure. It was precisely this inability to reconcile his sexuality with his spiritual beliefs that led him to leave the seminary as a young man. Now he felt there might be a way back into a spiritual life that did not exclude his eroticism.

Ward's spiritual journey intensified as he explored the importance of integrating the spiritual and the sexual in a personally more fulfilling, inclusive, and relevant notion of the sacred. Of the many readings he researched and shared with me, he was especially drawn to the Neoplatonists. The work of Plotinus in particular, as elaborated in Hines's (2004) book *Return to the Real*, was read, re-read, and adopted as a veritable manual for Ward's newly developing practice. He summarized Plotinus's disregard of the vulgar material world that obscures "God-realization" with the terse statement: "None of this matters." Naturally, this ultra-pragmatic stance became a challenge to our therapy as I understood and conducted it. If I made any interpretation that was not grounded in empirically verifiable experience, Ward dismissed it as mere "speculative chatter," more of the idealist self-serving rant he was at pains to eliminate through the meditation practice of quieting his mind.

Ward's study of Plotinus ultimately served as a prerequisite to an in-depth exploration of Gnosticism. He quickly consumed the writings of Pagels (1981), Rudolph (1987), and Meyer (2007), again, viewing these books more as instruction manuals for facilitating an effective spiritual practice than as historical studies. According to Ward, the Gnostics, unlike Plotinus, were not at pains to transcend the physical world, they located Divine Immanence within it. The unexpected effect of digesting the philosophy and aims of the Gnostic world view was a deeper, more passionate criticism of his Roman Catholic, experience-distant relationship with an imaginary mythic God. Eventually the insights of Plotinus and the Gnostics, as Ward understood them, cumulatively suggested that the Divine was located within Ward himself and could be accessed directly, even physically as an aspect of Self. This had a powerful revelatory impact on Ward as he ecstatically (and completely without irony) proclaimed that he felt a positive sense of self-possession and self-worth for the first time in his life.

As Ward's spiritual practice turned increasingly inward and became increasingly physical, he grew more convinced that the progress of his journey would be divinely sanctioned by an actual corollary sign from the Holy Ghost. Every day at lunch hour, he took his break in St. John the Baptist Church, a cathedral a few blocks from his office in midtown Manhattan. There he engaged in meditation and was deeply inspired and encouraged by the Shrine for Padre Pio who had been canonized as a saint in 1999. Of special importance for Ward was the presence of two relics exhibited inside reliquaries on the shrine. One was a white sock formerly owned and worn by Padre Pio, and the other was a glove worn by the saint (see Figure 1.1). On the saint's feast day, a fountain pen of Padre Pio was exhibited along with a photo of "the blessed one" writing a Christmas card with the same pen. Ward was delighted and inspired by the materiality of this shrine; indeed, this was good theater.

Ward became increasingly passionate at the therapeutic prospect of finally unifying several disparate strands of his life. His criticism of Christian "mythology" and bureaucracy; Christianity's (and his family's) dismissal of his homosexuality; his years on the New York art scene including the Warhol party circuit; his fondness for the historically layered, collage-effect of Italian architecture; Plotinus's views on the veil of materiality concealing sacred Immanence; and his recent, Gnostic-inspired, materially based identification with "the Divine" all blended and contributed to a self-styled religious practice that felt unequivocally meaningful. Inspired, Ward returned to his own artwork for the first time in over 30 years. Utilizing the skills he acquired over decades of making signs, Ward set out to create digital compositions of modern religious icons that expressed his political, philosophical, psychological, and artistic views (on the construction and nature of icons as distinguished from other signs, see Mitchell 1986 and Sebeok 1994).

The digital compositions were all constructed on his home computer using scanned and downloaded images from a wide diversity of sources: art history, architecture, pornography, toy catalogues, and so on. The iconic images are deliberately vulgar juxtapositions, collage-style, of sacred Christian images and modern pulp pornography and are strongly informed by Ward's liberating interpretation of Gnosticism. As though he were commenting directly on Ward's compositions, Bataille (1991a), in an affirming, analogous vein, remarked,

> The interest of this juxtaposition is augmented by the fact that the specific reactions of Gnosticism led to the representation of forms

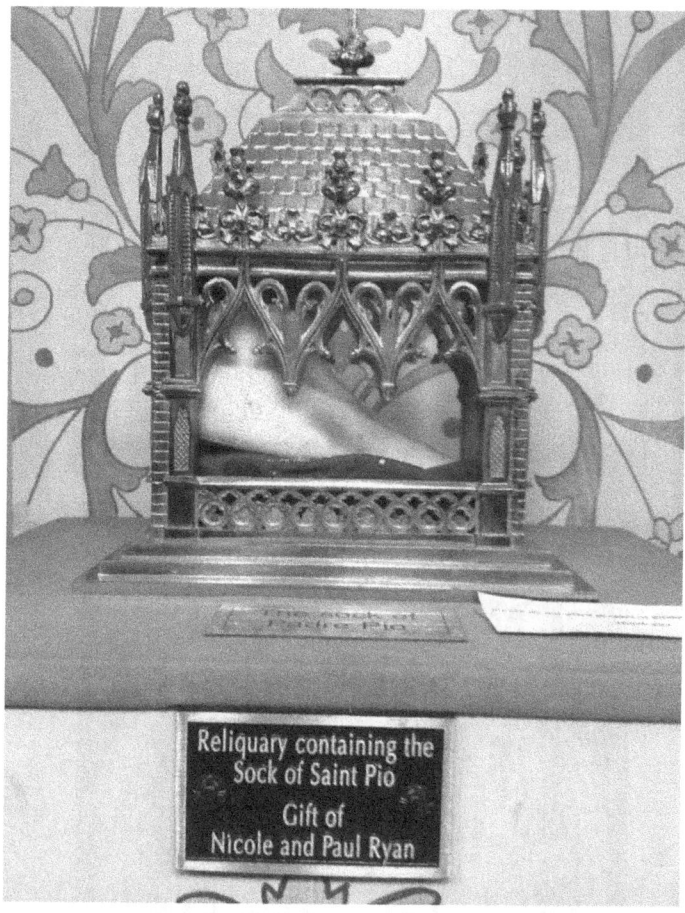

Figure 1.1 Padre Pio's sock reliquary.
Source: All photographs taken by the author.

radically contrary to the ancient academic style, to the representation of forms in which it is possible to see the image of this base matter that alone, by its incongruity and by an overwhelming lack of respect, permits the intellect to escape from the constraints of idealism.

51

Indeed, I experienced Ward's contemporary juxtapositions as graphic embellishments of the homogeneous/heterogeneous conflict underlying primitive sacred icons (Figures 1.2–1.6).

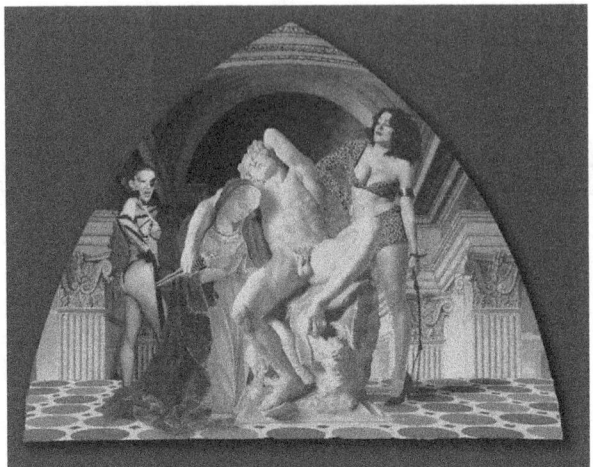

Figure 1.2 Pietà.

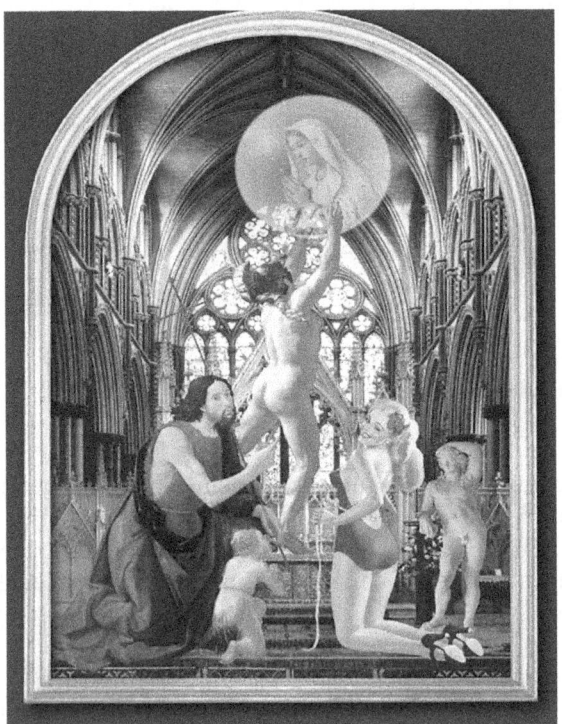

Figure 1.3 Hail the Madonna.

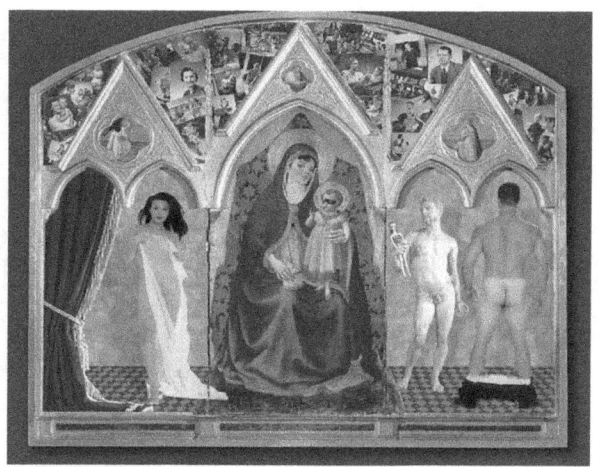

Figure 1.4 Triptych.

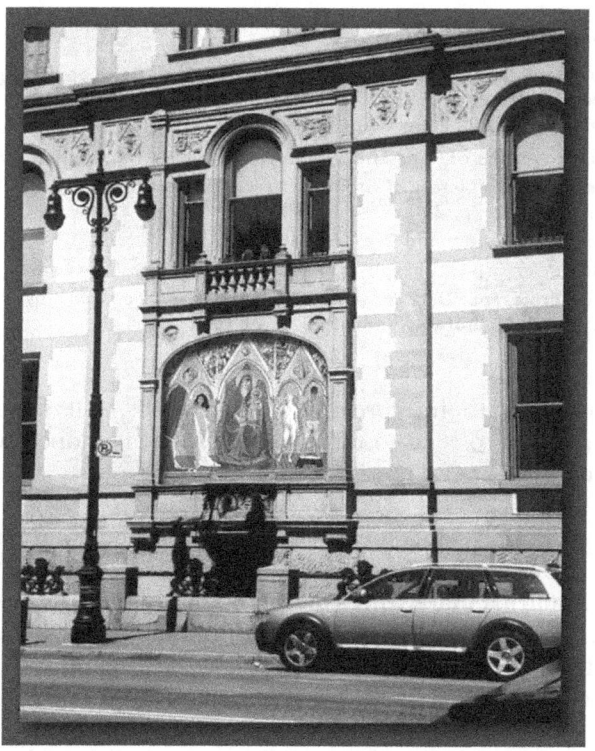

Figure 1.5 Triptych, in situ.

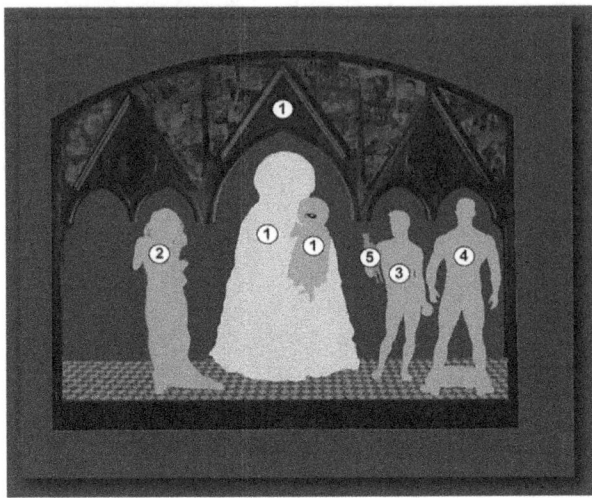

Figure 1.6 Triptych, references.

REFERENCES

1 Bartz, Gabriele, *Fra Angelico, Master's of Italian Art,* Sally Bald, ed. Cologne: Konemann Verlagsgesellschaft mbH, 1998, p. 15.
   Guido di Piero (Fra Angelico), "San Pietro Martire Triptych" (modified).
2 Mizuno, (photographs of Sung Hi Lee), *Playboy's Nudes,* (November 1999), p. 2.
3 Scalini Mario, ed. *The Library of Great Masters: Benvenuto Cellini,* New York: Riverside Book Company, 1995, p. 20.
   Baccio Bandinelli, "Adam and Eve", (modified).
4 Bull "Feelin Lucky", (photographs of Paul Carrigan), *Men* (December, 1999), p. 37.
5 Tosa Marco *Barbie, Four Decades of Fantasy, Fashion and Fun, tans,* by Linda M. Eklund. New York: Harry N. Abrams, Inc. 1998, p. 21.

Ward was loath to interpret his compositions, but he did write an accompanying text to send to those galleries that he hoped would exhibit them; it read,

> We are both body and spirit – sensuousness and transcendence. This duality of existence defines the essence of our humanity. It inspires the literature and art that realizes the mythology of life. Through mythology and art we attempt to comprehend our true nature ... [The] conceptual integration of the animal/divine dichotomy achieved through the transcendence of sex is an historic component of the duality of our human nature and is evident through literature and art ... Sexuality in Christian mythology develops a different symbolism ... [there] the ritual of sexuality, as expressed in classic mythology, devolves into an ascetic

virginity typified by the Madonna and an asexual Christ ... the [Christian] teachings tend to deny the most elemental part of our humanity with our connection to the divine. The modern view of body and spirit separates the sexual and the spiritual. In an historical context this division is a relatively recent phenomenon ... Could it be that the sacred is still present but perhaps hidden in the rituals of sex, whether in candle lit bedrooms, darkened theatres or on glowing computer screens?

In these compositions, icons from religious and secular traditions are juxtaposed in an attempt to reunite universal elements of mythology – the sacred and the profane. The digital combination of diverse images form an eclectic review of diverse periods, styles and techniques. They form, in a modern medium, a 21st century narrative expressing the integration of our cultural history and humanity.

When seen in a public context, the compositions assume an alternate significance. In relation to architecture, they have a completely different sense of scale – at once smaller and larger. The context evokes different questions of relevance and different historical references. In a modern sense, they become part of the landscape and are reduced to a decorative element.

As a reference, the compositions are reduced to abstract monochromatic forms. The experience is academic and cerebral. The bibliographic references expose the origins of the appropriated material. And in an academic format, they lay bare the intellectual pretensions of pretty pictures.

(personal manuscript, January 21, 2004)

As quickly as he began, Ward abruptly stopped producing any additional icons. Feeling just as he did with his employment dilemma, he simply could not tolerate the prospect of explaining and defending his work to others who would be either confused or critical. With this pessimistic forecast for his work's reception, and his weariness at the prospect of interpreting his compositions, Ward further withdrew. Around this time, he saw the film *Into Great Silence* (Groning 2005), a documentary of the Carthusian monks of the Grande Chartreuse, and became preoccupied with the silent routine of the monks' life. He began to research and visit monastic retreats as frequently as he could. At first, he took weekend excursions to the nearest retreat in Poughkeepsie, New York, but eventually felt it was too commercial and further expanded his search. This led to monastery retreat visits in California, the Southwest, and Europe before locating his favorite, the Desert House of Prayer (affectionately referred to as DHOP) in Tucson, Arizona.

Paralleling Ward's expanded geographic and theological range of interest, or perhaps in response to his renewed impulse to retreat, I began to experiment with the parameters of our psychotherapeutic relationship. In addition to our usual, conventional weekly office visits, I began to make annual "studio visits" to Ward in his Brooklyn home. During our four visits of this type, always in the summer when my schedule allowed, Ward and I spent hours viewing and discussing his artwork, the hundreds of photos he took at each retreat location, and the religious artifacts he began collecting. We were both self-consciously colluding around the notion that the spoken words and gestures of our usual meetings would be greatly enhanced by the actual visual and material experience of his photos, his self-constructed icons, as well as the tactile experience of his religious artifacts.

Of particular importance to Ward's increasing emphasis on material objects was his singular obsession with the crucifix. This sacred object with its symbolic dominance had both attracted and repelled Ward all his life. Without fully understanding why, Ward began to collect crucifixes from every location he visited. This gradually progressed to online acquisitions with Ward spending hundreds of dollars on eBay for more and more crucifixes. His criterion of selection was primarily aesthetic, but size was a consideration for proper display purposes. He had several boxes custom-made in order to contain and easily show his collection. However, the growing number of crucifixes soon exceeded the carrying capacity of all his boxes and he started lining the shelves of his home with them (see Figure 1.7). With each summer visit to Ward, I witnessed his home gradually transformed into a shrine (see Figure 1.8). It was as though the domestic excess of this particular material sign itself embodied a power that far surpassed its customary symbolic religious meaning, to say nothing of a reductionist Freudian interpretation of the crucifix as a phallus. Thus, a large part of my time with him there became devoted to sifting through – looking, touching, weighing, discussing – the various styles informing the sign of the cross; a fitting therapeutic activity integrating both the sacred and profane dimensions of Ward's interest insofar as "the cross affirms the primary relationship between the two worlds of the celestial and the earthly" (Cirlot 2002, 69).

As Ward turned 65 years old, his thoughts turned to retirement, leaving his job as a sign-maker, leaving Brooklyn and the steep financial cost of life in New York City, and facing the rest of his life fully devoted to developing his spiritual interests. After several considerations and months of research, Ward focused on Tucson, Arizona as his retirement destination and his final earthly home. It would be cheaper, near a cultural center (with close proximity to the University of Arizona), and of course, he'd be in close proximity to DHOP. For several months, Ward discussed Tucson as the land in the west where he would be fully realized, as though Tucson became symbolic of the fulfillment of Ward's journey.

Within weeks of settling on his plans to relocate, Ward was diagnosed with an exceptionally pernicious form of spinal cancer that quickly ravaged his body. Ward assured me that he was ready to die, he just didn't look forward to the process. Our last meetings in his home and in the hospital were dominated by his crying and howling due to extraordinary pain. His last request of me was that I arrange for him to have a very short haircut so

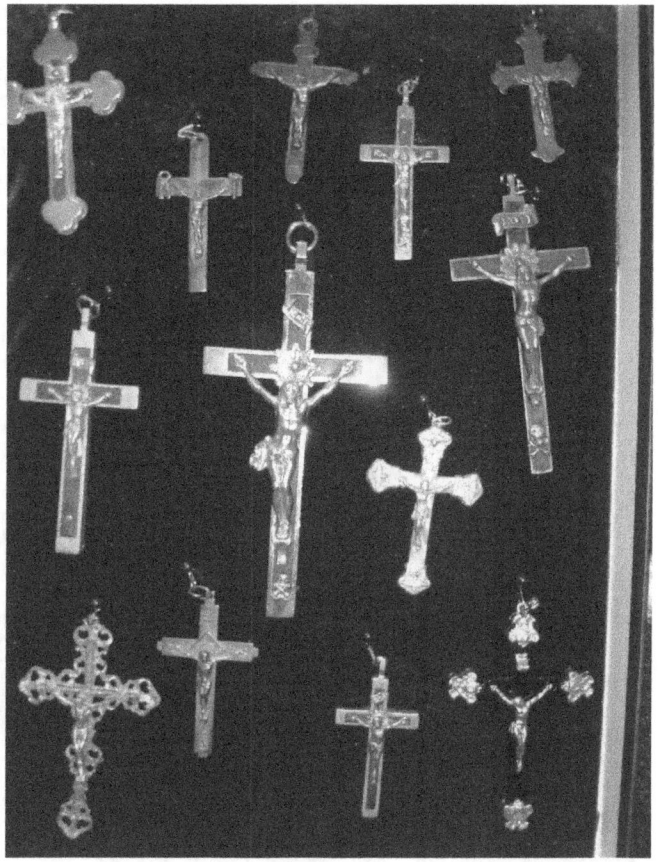

Figure 1.7 The growing number of crucifixes.

that the toll of the chemotherapy would be unnoticeable. However, it was too late for even the barber; within weeks of the cancer diagnosis, Ward was dead at age 66.

It is impossible for me not to think of Tucson as Ward's mantic metaphor for the land of the dead (as in Malinowski's 1954 depiction of the Trobriander's Tuma, or as the place "beyond" that parallels our own world, according to Canetti 1993, where the "double crowd" of the dead are waiting and watching). But Ward's photos, descriptions, and artifacts suggested otherwise. True to his embrace of Gnosticism, he denied the metaphoric displacement inherent in the Roman Catholic idealist notion of an afterlife right to the end. Ward was enthralled with the bone-dry materiality of Tucson, a sensual experience, as he described it, that was compatible with his self-styled asceticism. It was only the land of the dead to the extent that he knew he could disintegrate

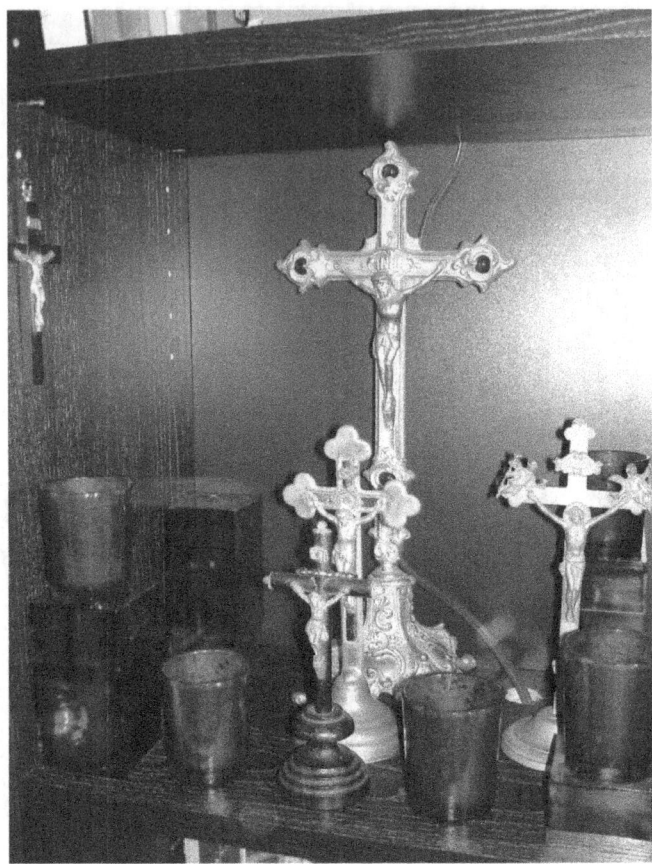

Figure 1.8 His home gradually transformed into a shrine.

there, in a fashion after all other living organisms, into formlessness and insignificance. As though acknowledging a final sign from this sign-maker, Bataille (1986) commented, "A dead body cannot be called nothing at all, but that object, that corpse, is stamped straight off with the sign 'nothing at all'" (57), or finally, in Ward's own words, "None of this matters."

Bibliography

American Disabilities Act – Architectural Barriers Act. *Current ABA Standards, Online Guidance*. Retrieved from www.access-board.gov/ada-aba/guide.htm.
Barthes, Roland. *Elements of Semiology*. Translated by Annette Lavers and Colin Smith. New York: Hill and Wang, 1994/1964.

Bataille, Georges. *Erotism: Death & Sensuality*. Translated by Mary Dalwood. San Francisco, CA: City Lights Books, 1986/1957.

Bataille, Georges. "Notes on the Foundation of a College of Sociology." In *The College of Sociology, 1937–39*, 3–5. Edited by Denis Hollier. Translated by Betsy Wing. Minneapolis, MN: University of Minnesota, 1988a/1937.

Bataille, Georges. "Attraction and Repulsion II: Social Structure." In *The College of Sociology, 1937–39*, 113–124. Edited by Denis Hollier. Translated by Betsy Wing. Minneapolis, MN: University of Minnesota Press, 1988b/1938.

Bataille Georges. "Base Materialism and Gnosticism." In *Visions of Excess: Selected Writings, 1927–1939*, 45–52. Edited and translated by Allan Stoekl. Minneapolis, MN: University of Minnesota Press, 1991a/1930.

Bataille, Georges. "The Psychological Structure of Fascism." In *Visions of Excess: Selected Writings, 1927–1939*, 137–160. Edited and translated by Allan Stoekl. Minneapolis, MN: University of Minnesota Press, 1991b/1933.

Baudrillard, Jean. *Symbolic Exchange and Death*. Translated by Iain H. Grant. London: Sage Publications, 1995/1976.

Benjamin, Walter 1936. "The Work of Art in the Age of Its Technological Reproducibility: Second Version." In *Walter Benjamin: Selected Writings, Volume 3, 1935–38*, 101–133. Edited by Howard Eiland and Michael W. Jennings. Translated by Edmund Jephcott, Howard Eiland, et al. Cambridge, MA: Belknap Press, 2002/1936.

Canetti, Elias. *Crowds and Power*. Translated by Carol Stewart. New York: Noonday Press, 1993.

Chatwin, Bruce. *The Songlines*. New York: Penguin Books, 1987.

Cirlot, Juan Eduardo. *A Dictionary of Symbols*. Mineola, NY: Dover Publications, 2002.

Douglas, Mary. *Purity and Danger*. London: Penguin Books, 1966.

Geertz, Clifford. "Religion." In *Magic, Witchcraft, and Religion: An Anthropological Study of the Supernatural*, 6–15. Edited by Arthur C. Lehmann and James E. Myers. Mountain View, CA: Mayfield Publishing, 1989.

Groning, Philip. *Into Great Silence*. Zeitgeist Films, 2005.

Hines, Brian. *Return to the One: Plotinus' Guide to God-Realization*. Salem, OR: Adrasteia Publishing, 2004.

Lévi-Strauss, Claude. *Introduction to the Work of Marcel Mauss*. Translated by Felicity Baker. London: Routledge & Kegan Paul, 1987.

Lynch, Kevin. *The Image of the City*. Cambridge, MA: MIT Press, 1960.

Malinowski, Bronisław. *Magic, Science, and Religion: And Other Essays*. Garden City, NY: Doubleday and Company, 1954.

McLuhan, Marshall. *Understanding Media: The Extensions of Man*. Cambridge, MA: MIT Press, 2002/1964.

Meyer, Marvin (ed.). *The Nag Hammadi Scriptures: The Revised and Updated Translation of Sacred Gnostic Texts*. Translated by the Coptic Gnostic Library Project of the Institute for Antiquity and Christianity of Claremont Graduate University. New York: HarperCollins Publishers, 2007.

Mitchell, W. J. T. *Iconology: Image, Text, Ideology*. Chicago, IL: The University of Chicago Press, 1986.

Oxford English Dictionary. English (US) London: Oxford University Press, 2014. Retrieved from www.oxforddictionaries.com/definition/american_english/sign.

Pagels, Elaine. *The Gnostic Gospels*. New York: Vintage Books, 1981.

Peirce, Charles S. "Division of Signs." In *Collected Papers*, 783138. Edited by Charles Hartshorne. Dublin, OH: OCLC, 1932/1897.

Rudolph, Kurt. *Gnosis: The Nature and History of Gnosticism*. Translated by Robert M. Wilson. San Francisco, CA: Harper & Row, 1987.

Saussure, Ferdinand de. *Course in General Linguistics*. Translated by Wade Baskin. New York: McGraw Hill Books, 1966/1915.

Sebeok, Thomas A. *Signs: An Introduction to Semiotics*. Toronto: University of Toronto Press, 1994.

Steinberg, Leo. *The Sexuality of Christ in Renaissance Art and in Modern Oblivion*. Chicago, IL: The University of Chicago Press, 1997.

Weber, Max. "Science as a Vocation." In *From Max Weber: Essays in Sociology*, 129–156. Edited by Hans H. Gerth and Charles Wright Mills. New York: Oxford University Press, 1958/1918.

Chapter 2

The distance between spending and spent

On manic consuming, hoarding, expending, and other visions of excess

> I never want to see you again … I despise you. Not just unprofessional, you're evil. First you seduced me and then wouldn't sleep with me. What possessed me to want to sleep with you, you cad? I've had many therapists but you have proven to be the worst … I should report you for the loser you are. Find another profession you son of a bitch!

With these words Judy terminated our treatment relationship, which had consisted of multiple 45-minute sessions each week continuously for ten years. Of course, this was not our first falling out, but over time her explosions grew more intense, more adamant, and more overtly threatening with an expressed intent to destroy.

My efforts to personally withstand these tirades led me to conceptualize them as evidence of manic depression, more conventionally referred to today as bipolar disorder. Indeed, this diagnosis had followed Judy from a young age. For her entire adult life, she experienced this label as deeply offensive, inaccurate, and stigmatizing – especially when she was "high"; conversely, she experienced the same classification as tragically accurate and hopeless when coming down off a high. So there existed a striking relationship between her frequent manic states and her rejection of the psychiatric nosology that classified this euphoria as pathological and dangerous.

By the time Judy and I met she had engaged and rejected the professional services of several mental health clinicians and had also tried and rejected several psychiatric mood stabilizing medications such as Lithium, Depakote, and Lamictal, to name but a few. At the outset of our work together she adamantly declared that she would no longer utilize mood stabilizing medication as part of her treatment. In fact, a condition upon commencing our work was that I would conduct the psychotherapy along classical psychoanalytic lines, perhaps a wish based on her idealized late father's career as a psychoanalyst. In other words, she insisted upon a "talking" procedure.

Judy's initial adamant rejection of any psychiatric attribution and accompanying medication (conventionally prescribed for mania) was continuously reiterated, despite or because of the apparently strong correlation between her behavior and the defining criteria of bipolar disorder as described in the Diagnostic and Statistical Manual of Mental Disorders, Fifth Edition of the American Psychiatric Association (DSM-5) (2013, 123–129):

The essential feature of a manic episode is a distinct period during which there is an abnormally, persistently elevated, expansive, or irritable mood and persistently increased activity or energy that is present for most of the day, nearly every day, for a period of at least one week (or any duration if hospitalization is necessary), accompanied by at least three additional symptoms from Criterion B.

Criterion B of either the Manic or Hypomanic Episode varieties of bipolar disorder consists of the following:

1 Inflated self-esteem or grandiosity.
2 Decreased need for sleep (e.g. feels rested after only three hours of sleep).
3 More talkative than usual or pressure to keep talking.
4 Flight of ideas or subjective experience that thoughts are racing.
5 Distractibility (i.e. attention too easily drawn to unimportant or irrelevant external stimuli), as reported or observed.
6 Increase in goal-directed activity (either socially, at work or school, or sexually) or psychomotor agitation (i.e. purposeless non-goal-directed activity).
7 Excessive involvement in activities that have a high potential for painful consequences (e.g. engaging in unrestrained buying sprees, sexual indiscretions, or foolish business investments).

124

While all of these criteria were predictably, persistently, and cyclically in evidence with Judy, I will focus on only the last point, that is, the excessive involvement in activities such as "unrestrained buying sprees"; this being especially pertinent to the development of the treatment as I understood it. During the history of our work together, her excessive buying included the impulsive purchase of a guitar and guitar lessons, a bicycle (rarely if ever used), dog-walking services, a professional office space (despite not having an active professional vocation), airline tickets, driving courses (though she had no car and never drove otherwise), extensive apartment renovations and furniture, jewelry, season subscription tickets to a variety of performances, multiple additional psychotherapists and a psychiatrist – the latter of whom she routinely visited concurrent with our treatment relationship, and so on. It is important to note that Judy spent prodigiously despite holding only part-time employment for nominal wages during most of our time working together. However, the greatest part of these shopping sprees was reserved for the purchase of gifts which were given continuously and seemingly indiscriminately to anyone in her social realm (including her dog). I was given all manner of items.

As per our agreement, in typical psychoanalytic fashion I initially attempted to work with the spending and gifting flings through the developmental experience of Judy's body. Freud (1908), Abraham (1927), and Ferenczi (1914) all suggested a derivative relationship between gifts and feces and described the anal character along with the fate of toilet training in general as fundamental to the attitude and behavior associated with presenting and receiving gifts. In this vein I assessed her need for my approval and blessing of her generosity as a veiled wish for praise over a good elimination. Yet regardless of how I framed my concern for her spending, I appeared to Judy and myself as withholding, overly parsimonious, and even envious of her carefree spending sprees. This perception of me as a killjoy would eventually and perhaps necessarily flourish into a major aspect of our relationship.

Buying and gifting material objects represented only one aspect of how Judy spent copiously without discrimination. After some time in treatment she discovered through a third party that I was divorced. This prompted a profuse and intense onslaught of appeals for a romantic liaison with me through poems, recorded music, prepared food items, and other gifts. Her openly stated intention, indeed her newly established purpose for being in treatment was to seduce me. While it is practically expected that a patient develops loving feelings toward his/her analyst (see Freud 1914 on erotic transference) and even encouraged and employed in the service of the treatment, any hint of colluding or acting on these feelings by the analyst is potentially traumatic. My failure to comply with Judy's wish to commence a romantic relationship had the surprising effect of invoking the memory of her father's abrupt death – a pivotal event in her twenties that shortly preceded the onset of her manic cycles. To the extent that my refusal to have sex with her foreclosed on a fantasy, it was reminiscent of the earlier loss and in turn triggered a compensatory manic high transcending the pain of that loss (see Freud 1917 on mania related to mourning and loss). Again, asserting my professional, ethical boundaries based on the Hippocratic Oath to "do no harm" simply felt to her like a cold-hearted rejection from a prudish stick-in-the-mud.

In deference to Judy's adamant demand that I not reduce her euphoric experience to another uncontrollable manic episode, I sought to focus on her dismay at having to give up such exalted and exuberant feelings; I empathized with the pain she endured in losing a loving relationship with her father, in losing her youth, in coming down from her highs, in leaving Paradise, so to speak; but all to no avail. She tolerated my dynamic interpretations, or perhaps more accurately, my failure to sanction her highs as legitimate experiences unto themselves, as well as she could yet she did not relent. Rather, the intensity and frequency of the gifts, poems, and songs (sometimes sung) increased.

Months and months of dozens and dozens of frustrating sessions left me questioning my need for Judy to change and behave differently, particularly as she insisted she was not endangering herself in any way and that the problem I wanted to "help" her with was my own. Was she correct, was my diagnosis driven by latent moral judgment? If so, it behooved me to identify and address the basis of my own moral values. Capitalist society, my society, spawns, inculcates, and demands its own moral code – one which equates conserving with cleanliness, asceticism, and a virtuous life, certainly a Puritanical code with regard to spending versus conserving. Moreover, it is a code in which the accumulation of capital is fundamentally equated with the accumulation of grace (Weber 1948; Tawney 1962). My endopsychic focus based on the psychiatric medical model of the DSM V had a moral tone to it; one that obfuscated the role of the socioeconomic and sociocultural contexts that are increasingly thought to play a crucial role in the etiology of manic-depression (see Jamison 1993; Martin 2007).

Suppose I was to expand the customary analytic inquiry into the patient's developmental history to include the normative historical context for ecstatic spending? In what world did Judy's behavior make sense? In order to understand the exceptional position of ecstatic spending in a larger social context I turned to the work of social theorist Georges Bataille. Referencing pre-capitalist societies, Bataille (1991b) introduced his "notion of expenditure." As Stoekl (2007) summarizes,

> The theory itself is quite straightforward: living organisms always, eventually, produce more than they need for simple survival and reproduction. Up to a certain point, their excess energy is channeled into expansion … but inevitably the expansion of a species comes against limits: pressure will be exerted against insurmountable barriers.
> 36

Regarding these limits, Bataille (1988, 30) states,

> life suffocates within limits that are too close; it aspires in manifold ways to an impossible growth; it releases a steady flow of excess resources, possibly involving large squanderings of energy. The limits of growth being reached, life, without being in a closed container, at least enters into ebullition. Without exploding, its extreme exuberance pours out in a movement always bordering on an explosion.

According to Bataille's own peculiar anthropological vision, these "limits of growth" are manifest both in the taboo systems general to our society as well as in my particular profession and this inevitable "pouring out" takes on the form of the taboo's transgression: "There exists no prohibition that cannot be transgressed. Often the transgression is permitted, often it is even prescribed" (Bataille 1986, 63).

Regarding the importance of this transgression, Bataille cites the historic example of the spectacular potlatch ceremony of the Northwest American Coast Kwakiutl community. This now-outlawed relic of pre-capitalist economic life occurred around changes in social status (e.g., weddings) and other events affecting two or more families – in short, around social change. The potlatch centrally featured a ceremonial establishment of rank and respect based on an exchange of goods, each one greater than the other, each "generous" gesture intended to defy the ability of the other to reciprocate. In other words, a warring with gifts.

> The behavior which was required of the chief was arrogant and tyrannical to a degree … The great social check that acted to keep his activity within limits they phrased as a moral tabu: the tabu on overdoing … Society set limits, though the limits seem to us fantastic.
>
> Benedict (1959, 195)

Indeed, Benedict characterizes the Kwakiutl as Dionysian as she describes the unmoved indifference of a chief setting his own home on fire in an extreme gesture of loss beyond reciprocation, thereby shaming his guests while retaining or acquiring the highest respect and social status (193).

With this pre-capitalist, pre-modern portrait of economic life, Bataille moves us beyond an individualistic, ethnocentric focus to a consideration of a universal process informing widely divergent behaviors across several cultures of our species, even affecting the ways in which we theorize ourselves. The Bataillean theoretical "explosion" inverted the capitalist emphasis on utilitarianism, accumulation, and conservation for preservation and survival with a perspective that privileges the non-utilitarian production of excess in order to spend. Thus, his theorizing subsumed and elucidated other cognate, previous theoretical notions. Specifically, Bataille's "ebullition" is derivative of the notion of "collective effervescence," a term coined by Émile Durkheim to describe a universal social pattern (in *The Elementary Forms of Religious Life* 1995; on this highly influential text for Bataille, see Richman 2002).

For Durkheim, collective effervescence was one aspect of a bipolar social pattern that, like the potlatch, characterized the ceremonies of pre-modern aboriginal life. Working from the ethnographies of early missionaries, he references, among others, the *corroboree*, an aboriginal nocturnal dance festival of the Warramunga tribe of Central Australia in which women are exchanged (Spencer and Gillen 1899, 96–97); and the *Jeraeil*, an aboriginal nocturnal dance festival of the Kurnai tribe of Southeast Australia in which boys are separated from their female relatives and initiated into manhood (Howitt 1904, 617). The first phase of these ceremonies given over to profane production, preparation, and economic activity "is generally of rather low intensity" (Durkheim 1995, 217); the other phase concerns the social gatherings for sacred ceremonial or religious purposes that are non-productive or noneconomic and would by contrast be considered as occurring at high intensity:

> The effervescence often becomes so intense that it leads to outlandish behavior; the passions unleashed are so torrential that nothing can hold them. People are so far outside the ordinary conditions of life, and so conscious of the fact, that they feel a certain need to set themselves above and beyond ordinary morality.
>
> 218

In the case of the corroboree this entailed what we would conventionally describe as excessive, licensed promiscuity accompanying the exchange of women.

Moreover, the potential "explosion" Bataille suggests may also be seen as synonymous with the "discharge" associated with crowds. Canetti (1993) states,

> The most important occurrence within the crowd is the *discharge*. Before this the crowd does not actually exist; it is the discharge which creates it. This is the moment when all who belong to the crowd get rid of their differences and feel equal … In that density, where there is scarcely any space between, and body presses against body, each man is as near the other as he is to himself; and an immense feeling of relief ensues. It is for the sake of this blessed moment, when no-one is greater or better than another, that people become a crowd.
>
> 17–18 (author's emphasis)

Bataille's (1991b) own examples of non-productive expenditure help to further elucidate the privileging of excess through the principle of loss. In addition to the aforementioned potlatch ceremony, he cites, "luxury, mourning, war, cults, the construction of sumptuary monuments, games, spectacles, arts, perverse sexual activity (i.e., deflected from genital finality) – all these represent activities which, at least in primitive circumstances, have no end beyond themselves" (118). However, the preeminent form of loss or discharge that a crowd can express is the act of sacrifice. Sacrifice is the penultimate form of gifting; it is a solution to the excessive surplus that has reached a limit to growth, it is the explosion. It is gifting propelled by "a certain power which forces them to circulate, to be given away" (Mauss 1967, 41); it is that particular type of discharge that serves equally as a "release" (Hubert and Mauss 1964, 32–33). Bataille elaborates,

> The problem posed is that of the expenditure of the surplus. We need to give away, lose, or destroy. But the gift would be senseless (and so we would never decide to give) if it did not take on the meaning of an acquisition. Hence *giving* must become *acquiring a power*. Gift-giving has the virtue of a surpassing of the subject who gives, but in exchange for the object given, the subject appropriates the surpassing: He regards his virtue, that which he had the capacity for, as an asset, as a *power* that he now possesses. He enriches himself with a contempt for riches, and what he proves to be miserly of is in fact his generosity.
>
> 69 (1988; author's emphases)

The loss implied in giving becomes an acquisition of power, a power to surpass the subject, a power that is proportionate to the *non-productive* value of the gift given, an irredeemable loss. From this vantage point Judy may now be reconsidered – no longer as merely difficult and self-destructive, but perhaps as determined to *transgress* the taboo structure that manifested as this therapist's therapeutic "frame" (see Langs 1990); as her effort to divest, spend, or lose herself thereby acquiring a peculiar type of power (over the reductionist and pejorative appellation of psychiatric patient). Similar arguments could be made for the purging of bulimics, the hair-pulling of trichotillomania, cutting or self-mutilation, and even overt suicidal behavior. What we have labelled masochism, generally speaking, reads differently within the general economy of Bataille when compared to what Holt (1989) describes as the closed and resolved hydraulic system of Freud. The general economy suggests a different system with a different dynamic – collect to spend; a different type of collecting, but especially those varieties of collecting only weakly rationalized as utilitarian when actually, ultimately, the collecting is *in order to* spend.

Again, the case of the aforementioned potlatch ceremony is an instructive comparative precursor to modern expressions of non-productive expenditure: "The accumulation of everything needed for the ceremony could take from one to four years" (Kan 1989, 43);

> Many of these were material things, named house-posts and spoons and heraldic crests, but the greater number were immaterial possessions, names, myths, songs, and privileges which were the great boast of a man of wealth. All these prerogatives ... were owned for the time by an individual who singly and exclusively exercised the rights which they conveyed. The greatest of these prerogatives, and the basis of all others, were the nobility titles.
>
> Benedict (1959, 183)

Every Kwakiutl individual entered this economic system from the moment they were given a name as a baby. Throughout life and through several potlatch ceremonies marking individual and social growth through all of life's transitions, "A person of any importance changed names as snakes changed their skins" (185). Although characterized by a different, pre-capitalist notion of property and wealth, the potlatch successfully functioned as "a validator of status [and] a distribution of property" (Suttles 1991, 105). Above all, it was *circulatory*. Through it, religious and economic life was integrated. And within this circulatory potlatch ceremonial system the driving force of sacred expenditure was contingent on a Kwakiutl version of hoarding, the result of what Durkheim referred to as the profane life of production.

The Fifth Edition of the DSM issued in 2013 establishes hoarding as a formal psychiatric diagnosis for the first time. It reads,

> The essential feature of hoarding disorder is persistent difficulties discarding or parting with possessions, *regardless of their actual value* ... The main reasons given for these difficulties are the *perceived utility* or aesthetic value of the items or strong sentimental attachment to the possessions ... Some individuals feel responsible for the fate of their possessions and often go to great lengths to avoid being wasteful ... virtually any item can be saved. The nature of items is not limited to possessions that most other people would define as useless or of limited value ... *Approximately 80–90% of individuals with hoarding disorder display excessive acquisition.* The most frequent form of excessive acquisition is *buying* ... Individuals with hoarding disorder typically experience distress if they are unable to or are prevented from acquiring items.
>
> 248 (emphasis added)

Hoarding is one side of the bipolar quality of a general economy affecting all organic life. Considered alone, it is the result of a singular focus on productivity despite Bataille's claim that

> Human activity is not entirely reducible to processes of production and conservation, and consumption must be divided into two parts ... the minimum necessary for the conservation of life and the continuation of the individual's productive activity in a given society [and] so-called unproductive expenditure.
>
> 1991b, 118

Without its complementary expenditure, hoarding, the *sine qua non* action of capitalism, ironically assumes a character now thought to be pathological.

However, more than a sickness of collecting, the hoarder suffers from an obsession with utility that doubles as a nearly phobic regard for expenditure.

> This material utility is limited to acquisition (in practice, to production) and to the conservation of goods … But even when he does not spare himself and destroys himself while making allowances for nothing, the most lucid man will understand nothing, or imagine himself sick; he is incapable of a *utilitarian* justification for his actions, and it does not occur to him that a human society can have, just as he does, an *interest* in considerable losses, in catastrophes that, *while conforming to well-defined needs*, provoke tumultuous depressions, crises of dread, and, in the final analysis, a certain orgiastic state.
>
> 116–117 (author's emphases)

Hence, effective clinical treatment involves the resolution of this economic/ psychological constipation through a purgative cure of non-productive or *useless* spending (see the last five minutes of every episode of the reality show Hoarding: Buried Alive). With a change in accent, this portends a newly imagined potential for capitalistic investment *and* divestment; for acquiring *and* charitable giving or tithing; for giving as a "therapeutic" sacrifice, as with the "turning it over to a higher power" that purportedly liberates the addict from the buying and consuming of substances; and also for psychoanalysis.

Although I have limited myself to the suggested contrast between a treatment conducted along classically Freudian analytic lines (as per the patient's request) and a Bataillean perspective of privileging notions of excess, psychoanalysis in any of its early or late permutations does not, by definition, escape the vagaries of a closed economy. Its hope for the future lies in its transgressive potential, once so important in its early establishment though now reduced, at best, to serving productive ends as a minor player in a growing mental health training industry (for a discussion of transgression as a foundational aspect of ressentiment in psychoanalysis see Buse 2006). Psychoanalysts must recognize, as Bataille did, that

> the Copernican revolution which Freud thought he was inaugurating, by showing that the human ego is not even master in its own house, is not complete until the human ego is forced to admit another master, the Dionysian principle of excess.
>
> Brown (1990, 183)

Judy's excessive buying and gifting, drinking binges, and explosive expressions of rage and love are unmitigated expressions of this bipolar quality of existence; a survival of a long-forgotten life cycle that, activated by trauma and early loss, reemerged undomesticated and unfit for a society that shamefully forbids and hides waste. In our closed economic and moral system that emphasizes redemption through productive usefulness, "the necessity of throwing oneself *out of oneself* remains the psychological or physiological mechanism that in certain cases can have no other end than death" (Bataille 1991a, 67). Ultimately, the most extreme act of love, beyond sexual union, was for Judy to annihilate me, to sacrifice our relationship and decimate us, our relationship, her view of treatment, her learned conventional notions of health and mental health, as well as her own previous positive regard for me (whether this be referred to as attachment, erotic transference, or love) all in one fell swoop.

In conclusion, I am left alone, cut off from any hope of reciprocity, writing and trying to get "closure" through a rational explanation that would redeem the months and years of passion and rancor that characterized our relationship – an exercise that will prove futile until I too can "surpass the subject."

Bibliography

Abraham, Karl. "Contributions to the Theory of Anal Character." In *Selected Papers on Psychoanalysis*, 370–392. Translated by Douglas Bryan and Alix Strachey. New York: Brunner/Mazel, 1927.

American Psychiatric Association. *Diagnostic and Statistical Manual of Mental Disorders, 5th Edition, DSM-5*. Washington, DC: American Psychiatric Publishing, 2013.

Bataille, Georges. *Erotism: Death & Sensuality*. Translated by Mary Dalwood. San Francisco, CA: City Lights Books, 1986.

Bataille, Georges. *The Accursed Share, Vol. 1*. Translated by Robert Hurley. New York: Zone Books, 1988.

Bataille, Georges. "Sacrificial Mutilation and the Severed Ear of Vincent Van Gogh." In *Visions of Excess, Selected Writings, 1927–1939*, 61–72. Edited and translated by Allan Stoekl. Minneapolis, MN: University of Minnesota Press, 1991a/1930.

Bataille Georges. "The Notion of Expenditure." In *Visions of Excess, Selected Writings, 1927–1939*, 116–129. Edited and translated by Allan Stoekl. Minneapolis, MN: University of Minnesota Press, 1991b/1933.

Benedict, Ruth. *Patterns of Culture*. Boston, MA: Houghton Mifflin Company, 1959.

Brown, Norman O. "Dionysus in 1990." In *Apocalypse and/or Metamorphosis*, 179–200. Edited by Norman O. Brown. Berkeley, CA: University of California Press, 1990.

Buse, William. "Toward a Genealogy of Psychoanalysis." In *The Psychoanalytic Review*, 521–539. Vol. 93 (4), August 2006.

Canetti, Elias. *Crowds and Power*. Translated by Carol Stewart. New York: Noonday Press, 1993.

Durkheim, Émile. *The Elementary Forms of Religious Life*. Translated by Karen E. Fields. New York: Free Press, 1995/1912.

Ferenczi, Sandor (1914). "The Ontogenesis of the Interest in Money." In *First Contributions to Psychoanalysis*, 319–331. Translated and edited by Ernest Jones. New York: Brunner Mazel, 1980/1914.

Freud, Sigmund. "Character and Anal Erotism." In *The Standard Edition of the Complete Psychological Works of Sigmund Freud, Volume IX*, 167–176. Edited and translated by James Strachey. London: Hogarth Press, 1959/1908.

Freud, Sigmund. "Observations on Transference-Love: Further Recommendations on the Technique of Psychoanalysis, III." In *The Standard Edition of the Complete Psychological Works of Sigmund Freud. Volume XII*, 157–171. Edited and translated by James Strachey. London: Hogarth Press, 1958/1914.

Freud, Sigmund. "Mourning and Melancholia." In *The Standard Edition of the Complete Psychological Works of Sigmund Freud, Volume XIV*, 237–258. Edited and translated by James Stachey. London: Hogarth Press, 1957/1917.

Hoarding: Buried Alive. Silver Spring, MD: The Learning Channel, 2014.

Holt, Robert R. *Freud Reappraised: A Fresh Look at Psychoanalytic Theory*. New York: Guilford Press, 1989.

Howitt, Alfred William. *The Native Tribes of South East Australia*. London: Macmillan and Company, 1904.

Hubert, Henri and Marcel Mauss. *Sacrifice: Its Nature and Function*. Translated by W. D. Halls. Chicago, IL: The University of Chicago Press, 1964.

Jamison, Kay Redfield. *Touched with Fire: Manic Depressive Illness and the Artistic Temperament*. New York: Free Press, 1993.

Kan, Sergei. *Symbolic Immortality: The Tlingit Potlatch of the Nineteenth Century*. Washington, DC: Smithsonian University Press, 1989.

Langs, Robert. *The Therapeutic Environment*. New York: Jason Aronson, 1990.

Martin, Emily. *Bipolar Expeditions: Mania and Depression in American Culture*. Princeton, NJ: Princeton University Press, 2007.

Mauss, Marcel. *The Gift: Forms and Functions of Exchange in Archaic Societies*. Translated by Ian Cunnison. New York: W. W. Norton & Company, 1967/1925.

Richman, Michele H. *Sacred Revolutions: Durkheim and the Collège de Sociologie*. Minneapolis, MN: University of Minnesota Press, 2002.

Spencer, Baldwin and F. G. Gillen. *The Native Tribes of Central Australia*. London: Macmillan and Company, 1899.

Stoekl, Allan. *Bataille's Peak: Energy, Religion, and Post-Sustainability*. Minneapolis, MN: University of Minnesota Press, 2007.

Suttles, Wayne. "Streams of Property, Armor of Wealth: The Traditional Kwakiutl Potlatch." In *Chiefly Feasts: The Enduring Kwakiutl Potlatch*, 71–134. Edited by Aldona Jonaitis. Seattle, WA: University of Washington Press, 1991.

Tawney, Richard Henry "Harry." *Religion and the Rise of Capitalism: A Historical Study*. Gloucester: Peter Smith, 1962.

Weber, Max. *The Protestant Ethic and the Spirit of Capitalism*. Translated by Talcott Parsons. New York: Charles Scribner's Sons, 1948.

Chapter 3

The other kind of laughter

> What matters to me insofar as I speak of laughter is situating it at that point of slippage which leads to that particular experience, the laughter which becomes divine insofar as it can be one's laughter at witnessing the failure of a tragic nature.
>
> Bataille (1953, 97)

No training and analysis, nor years of mortification and rigorous self-recrimination, have eradicated the embarrassing propensity to laugh in the face of abject failure. I have long accepted the possibility of appearing inappropriate at grim news and funerals. (It's not that these events are funny, but ...). In fact, these disruptions had become so predictable as to be somewhat controllable, like the hiccups. That is, until I met Lester.

Lester contacted me, complaining of unrelenting depression. We met for years (maybe it was only months), trudging through our weekly monotonous meetings, always despairing, always hopeless. Through my fog-like stupor, I gathered that Lester was as unforgiving of humans as he was idealizing of animals, especially dolphins. One day, long after his wariness of me had seeped into my weariness of him, I blurted out, "Let's go see a dolphin"! This desperate outburst startled us both. Soon after, we were sitting nervously together on the D train heading toward the Coney Island aquarium. He looked out the window and described his Brooklyn. Each familiar stop evoked another memory of the betrayal and injury that slowly twisted him into the anti-humanist he is today.

The conversation turned to dolphins. A great deal of research had been published. Dolphins possessed mythological importance in prehistory (Glueck 1965; McIntyre 1974); are known to have a very large cranial capacity with exceptional intelligence (Lilly 1971; Brown 1979); are capable of "thought-transfer" (Robson 1988); are known to heal autistic youths after extensive aquatic interaction (St. John 1991); and are believed to be sexually prodigious (Norris 1993; Slater 1994). Dolphin researchers are often pulled into fully mutual relationships with dolphins. Why, one researcher who

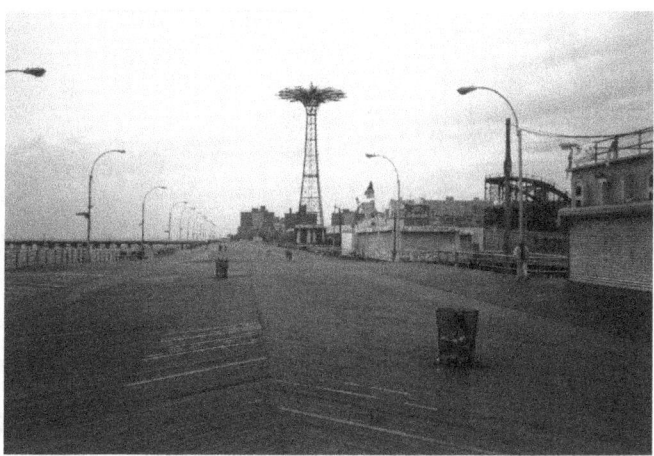

Figure 3.1 The Coney Island boardwalk.
Source: All photographs taken by the author.

worked with a single dolphin for years went so far as to stimulate the lonely mammal into ... we arrived at Coney Island.

After disembarking the train we headed for the boardwalk (see Figure 3.1). In its heyday, "Coney Island was necessarily an imperfect Feast of Fools, an institutionalized bacchanal" (Kasson 1995, 105). Now only the "profane illumination" of this once grand funfair remained (Benjamin 1999, 209). Yet somehow, we still felt a surprising sense of anticipation as we approached and entered the ruins of this place, why?

> Funfairs mean a break in the daily routine, in the exacting discipline of working life. They bring about an easing-off of the strict rules governing the life of society ... Expressed in psychological terms, this means that the environment not only tolerates aggressiveness and destructiveness and offers opportunities for them, but also, in a way, rejoices with the individual in its own destruction.
>
> Balint (1959, 19–21)

Lester showed me one of the attractions familiar from his early childhood visits here (see Figure 3.2). When we arrived at the aquarium, we were told the dolphins were moved to Florida while a new exhibition tank was being prepared. (The sharks were our consolation).

Overcome with stimulation, both internal and external, from the past as well as the present, Lester paused beneath the boardwalk for a cigarette (see Figure 3.3).

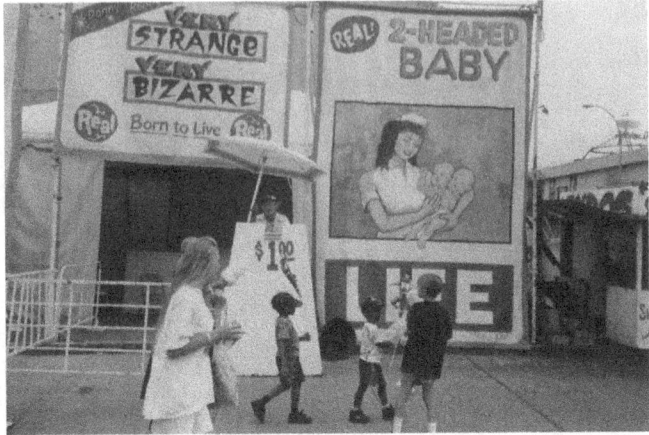

Figure 3.2 One of the attractions.

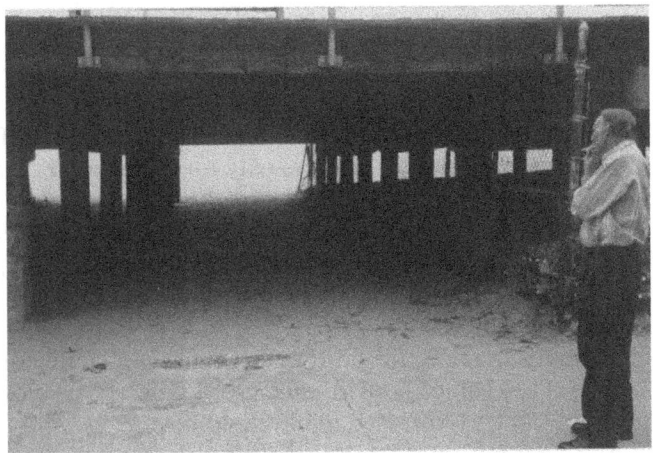

Figure 3.3 Lester paused beneath the boardwalk for a cigarette.

We went on more trips after this: back to the aquarium, to the Central Park zoo, and so on. Each journey's goal was Lester's trial identification with an animal, primarily fish or birds. Although Lester seemed less depressed, he became anxious as I grew increasingly enthusiastic about our trips. He began qualifying his beliefs about human-animal relationships and expressed concern about my mental health – I was either patronizing him or I was "sick" too. Lester's uneasiness reached its apex during our visit to a conference on "The Human Mimicry of Bird Sound" at the American Museum of Natural History. There, in the middle of an animated discussion with several avid ornithologists, Lester suddenly exclaimed, "we're all just a bunch of nuts, aren't we?" (This provoked the opposite of laughter). The group lowered their eyes, grew silent, and went home.

Lester descended back into the morass. On his insistence, we stopped our trips and resumed the safe and predictable cadence of our previous meetings, now more hopeless than ever, given our joint sense of failure. Long silences followed; our eyes rarely met. After one particularly bleak encounter, Lester slowly left the room shaking his head (in disbelief? in disgust?). As I sat down and looked out into space, I heard a sound coming from outside. It was so faint that, for a second, I thought I was dreaming. It sounded like a crow cawing in my bathroom. The mournful but resounding cry bounced off the tiled walls, creating a slight echo. Like a crow flying low in a canyon. (That's not a crow, that's Lester in the bathroom! Lester is out there cawing in the bathroom!) An equally resounding sound erupted below my neck and issued forth from my open mouth. A laugh as long as it was loud. Not a laughter born of resentment, fear, or false mutual assurance. And it's not that this was in the least bit funny, but oh, how I enjoyed this other kind of laughter.

Bibliography

Balint, Michael. *Thrills and Regressions.* New York: International Universities Press, 1959.

Bataille, Georges. "Un-knowing: Laughter and Tears." In *October*, 89–102. Vol. 36, Spring, 1986/1953.

Benjamin, Walter. "Surrealism: The Last Snapshot of the European Intelligentsia." In *Walter Benjamin, Selected Writings, Volume 2: 1927–1934*, 207–221. Edited by Michael W. Jennings, Howard Eiland, and Gary Smith. Translated by Rodney Livingstone and others. Cambridge, MA: Belknap Press, 1999/1929.

Brown, Robin. *The Lure of the Dolphin.* New York: Avalon Books, 1979.

Glueck, Nelson. *Deities and Dolphins: The Story of the Nabataeans.* New York: Farrar, Straus and Giroux, 1965.

Kasson, John F. *Amusing the Million. Coney Island at the Turn of the Century.* New York: Hill & Wang, 1995.

Lilly, John C. *The Mind of the Dolphin: A Nonhuman Intelligence.* New York: Avon Books, 1971.

McIntyre, Joan. *Mind in the Waters: A Book to Celebrate the Consciousness of Whales and Dolphins.* New York: Charles Scribner's Sons, 1974.

Norris, Kenneth S. *Dolphin Days: The Life and Times of the Spinner Dolphin.* New York: Avon Books, 1993.

Robson, Frank. *Pictures in the Dolphin Mind.* Dobbs Ferry, NY: Sheridan House, 1988.

Slater, Candace. *Dance of the Dolphin: Transformation and Disenchantment in the Amazonian Imagination.* Chicago, IL: The University of Chicago Press, 1994.

St. John, Patricia. *The Secret Language of Dolphins.* New York: Summit Books, 1991.

Chapter 4

Recovery

Wendy, a self-proclaimed "biker chick" from Perth, Australia, had stopped drinking. She had stopped using heroin too. The only vice she held onto was her Parliament Lights, which she smoked with ritual regularity from the time she woke up until she went to bed. Without alcohol, she no longer knew how to socialize, so she isolated and waited every evening until it was time to sleep, wake, and go back to her corporate job as an administrative assistant. After a while of this, she contacted me and said she wanted help regaining her confidence for something resembling a social life. With time I realized that the "something resembling a social life" would be our relationship. She scorned the mention of Alcoholics Anonymous, particularly its "higher power," and kept her former drinking buddies at bay. She emphatically declared that she would rather set the terms of her own "recovery."

After a couple of years in treatment relating tales that vacillated between the good old hell-raising days in Australia and her anxiety-ridden days behind a desk in midtown Manhattan, there came a sudden, shocking break in our routine. She was diagnosed with Stage 4 terminal lung cancer during a routine medical visit. While she underwent tests in a midtown hospital, I said I'd visit and she requested two roast beef sandwiches, both with mustard and mayonnaise. She accepted the sandwiches but dismissed my concern: "Don't get your tits in a tangle mate!" Later she came back home to her humble apartment in Hell's Kitchen where I went to visit her again. I asked her where things stood with her health. She told me that her doctor advised her to "get your affairs in order" and so she did. She proceeded to show me, with some pride, how she taped the names of her friends on each of her worldly possessions so that, in lieu of a will, everyone would possess something of her in perpetuity. She then informed me, without looking in my eyes, that her sobriety was over, there was no longer any point. She transgressed her self-imposed abstinence, made the forbidden calls, and quickly resumed her previous heroin and alcohol consumption. In no time at all, she recovered the biker chick.

I went to see Wendy one last time at the Memorial Sloan Kettering Hospital on the Upper East Side of Manhattan, which specializes in cancer treatment. As I emerged from a cab on York Avenue, I was taken aback to see her standing at the threshold of the entrance in her hospital gown and slippers: gaunt, pale and defiant, her right hand grasping the portable intravenous pole that held, in suspension, the medicine drip that looped down into a vein in her arm, her left hand holding a burning Parliament Light. There she stood sentinel, radiating all the splendor of Charon at the river Styx ... "as everything that can be seen as sacred, divine, or marvelous ... [like] a half-decomposed cadaver fleeing through the night in a luminous shroud" (Bataille 1991, 94).

Bibliography

Bataille, Georges. "The Use Value of D. A. F. Sade (An Open Letter to My Current Comrades)." In *Visions of Excess: Selected Writings, 1927–1939*, 91–102. Edited and translated by Allan Stoekl. Minneapolis, MN: University of Minnesota Press, 1991/1930.

Chapter 5

Excremental journey

Waste is allotropical. Its material quality is variously identifiable in either verb, noun, or adjective form, whether we consider it as action, object, or attribute. A glance at the etymological roots of the word "waste" reveals that it derives from a cognate group of terms: *vacancy/vacant/vacate/evacuate*. Partridge (1959) examines its early forms:

> Here we have three Latin words, *uacare*, to be empty, hence vacant or unoccupied, *uanus*, empty, emptied (of what was there), hence hollow, without substance, hence vain, and *usatus*, ravaged, desolate (also ravaging, desolating, devastating), hence uncultivated, desert ... akin to Latin *uastus* are old high German *wuosti*, middle high German *wuete*, German *wust*, old Frisian *wost*, old English *weste*, which, especially the last, have strongly influenced the passage of the English adjective *waste*.
>
> 756–757 (author's emphases)

The often-overlooked importance of waste in human life was a central concern of social theorist Georges Bataille (1991j, 23): "Man is not just the separate being that contends with the living world and with other men for his share of resources. The general movement of exudation (of waste) of living matter impels him, and he cannot stop it." For Bataille, the isomorphic social quality of all forms of waste is non-productive uselessness. Insofar as an object or action is not essential for the reproduction of human existence, it falls under the domain of waste. Bataille variously identified waste with surplus, the accursed, the heterogenous, the sacred, and excrement. It is this non-productive, useless character of waste that enabled Bataille (1991h) to equate the most esteemed objects of luxury with feces and excrement, an unconscious equation in human psychology well established by psychoanalysts (see Abraham 1927; Freud 1959; Ferenczi 1980b). From there, Bataille (1991h) addressed the common psychoanalytic equation of gifts with feces: "In unconscious forms, such as those described by psychoanalysis, [the gift] symbolizes excrement" (122) but he then extends it, accentuating the loss at stake in the gifting/excreting act: "The gift must be considered as a loss and thus as a partial destruction, since the desire to destroy is in part transferred onto the recipient [and] is linked to death" (122). Bataille's inquiry into this loss through the act of personal or social expenditure of gifting ranges from examinations of Van Gogh's auto-mutilation (1991e) to the Kwakiutl potlatch ceremony (1991j) to Aztec human sacrifice (1991j).

An early illustration of this sense of non-productive loss through expenditure is depicted in Bataille's (1987) novel *The Story of the Eye*. The enucleation of an eye at the center of the story becomes the (literally and figuratively) untethered object of waste that fulfills the definition of the sacred for Bataille and others – as "matter out of place" (Douglas 1970, 48) or "matter in the wrong place" (Freud 1959, 173). Barthes (1992, 239) commented on Bataille's preoccupation with the fate of this untethered object:

> How can an object have a story? No doubt it can pass from hand to hand [as anthropologically described by Mauss (1967); and Malinowski (1961)] … it can also pass from image to image [see Benjamin (2003)], so that its story is that of a migration, the cycle of the avatars it traverses far from its original being, according to the tendency of a certain imagination which distorts yet does not discard it.

Barthes focuses on Bataille's particular blend of metaphor and metonymy as he traces the vicissitudes of the untethered eye; metonymy here referring to the continuous, contiguous sequence of the eye's journey (Evans 1996, 113). Borrowing Barthes's critical distinction, we can say that while the gift metaphor in all its variety represents excrement, the metonymic action of gifting results in displacement, destruction, and loss, especially the loss of any hitherto association with useful function. As Barthes (1992) points out, "For Bataille, what matters is to traverse the vacillation of several objects … so that they exchange the functions of the obscene and those of substance" (246). In other words, vacated of its customary function, the object becomes a free-floating signifier holding all the potential this convulsive rupture portends: elimination, expulsion, eruption, exudation, ebullition, effervescence, explosion, expenditure, evacuation, eviction, ejaculation, expiation, and so on. Thus the excremental object of metaphor can travel, as Kussel (1976, 117), following Barthes, following Bataille, notes, from "the anus to the mouth to the eye."

We have all been on this journey before, not only as it pertains to the non-productive, useless objects metaphorically and metonymically strung together in our individual lives but on a societal level as well. Canetti (1993) famously describes the processes of discharge, destruction, and eruption we experience as objects ourselves within open and closed crowds. Thus, all of these actions were available as cultural possibilities, either consciously or unconsciously, to the mind and body of a patient seeking catharsis/discharge through psychotherapy with me.

My first impressions of Sam were non-verbal. He strode in short steps into my office, his gait stifled by his obesity. Although he stood at about five feet, seven inches tall he appeared shorter due to his weight of at least 300 pounds. He was so immense that, aside from his difficulty ambulating and breathing, his facial expressions were constrained by the puffiness of the fat held in his facial tissue. His clothes were too tight and disheveled which seemed to betray a marked lack of regard for his own appearance. Or rather, quite possibly, as I came to discover, he made exactly the impression he intended.

He seemed young, even younger than his stated 24 years. This might be because he spoke in a somewhat self-ashamed manner, as would a schoolboy caught for truancy. The one remarkably dissonant feature of his presentation was a twinkle in his eye that seemed to indicate that he was waiting for me to "get the joke." I understood quickly that my ability to get in on the joke would be pivotal to forming a good working alliance with him (Greenson 1979).

I learned that Sam was the only child, adopted, of an older Jewish couple who operated a wholesale fur trade in the fashion district of New York City. Sam lived with his parents in an affluent NY suburb and commuted with them to their shop each morning where he worked with them for a nominal wage. While the family was not religiously orthodox in practice, his parents' Jewish identity was evidently very important to them. Sam informed me that he was constantly enmeshed in bickering with his father all day, every day, due to his unavoidable tendency to tease his father for his heavy Yiddish accent and his recognizably common Jewish (Ashkenazi) name. Scott was at a complete loss or simply refused to explain to me why he insisted on teasing his father. However, whenever he spoke of the teasing, his eyes twinkled, he blushed, and he laughed.

From the outset, Sam created a diagnostic impression akin to a "dissocial" adolescent (Aichhorn 1974) with "antisocial tendencies" (Winnicott 1975), or, put simply, a "problem child" (Adler 1964). His lack of self-insight was striking, particularly in light of his extensive history in treatment throughout his childhood with a series of psychotherapists, always at his parents' insistence. In response to my direct questioning he stated, albeit unconvincingly, that this time it was he who wanted to be in treatment and that he was not just appeasing his parents. He reluctantly revealed that his last effort at treatment, in a clinic near his parents' home, ended with him being summarily discharged and pronounced by his psychotherapist as a "hopeless case." Again, the twinkle, the blush, and the laugh. I decided to follow his non-verbal cues and get the history behind his gleeful exasperation of others, including this most recent emphatic discharge.

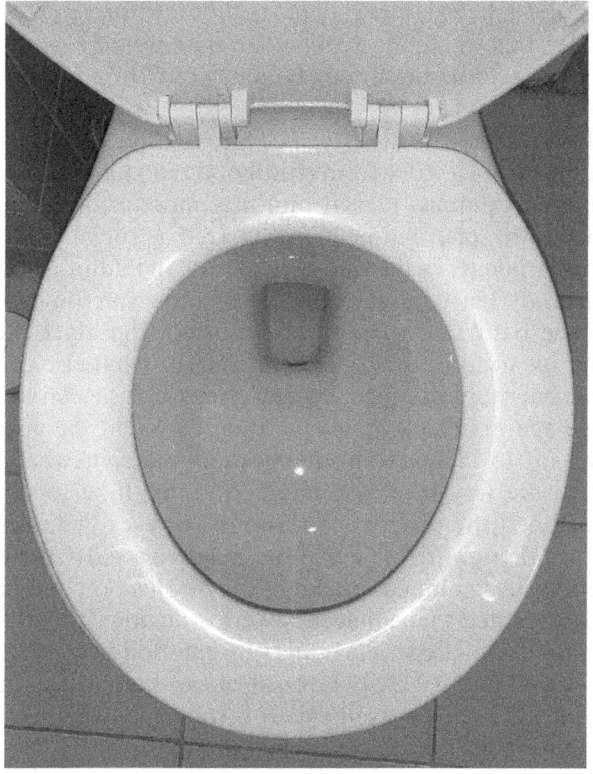

Figure 5.1 Toilet.
Source: All photographs taken by the author.

Sam's earliest memory of problems with others went back to childhood when he was seven years old. After sitting yet again for another boring, extended weekly Shabbos service with his parents on a Saturday afternoon he felt an impulse to act. When no one was looking he slipped into the room where the Rabbi kept his personal items, grabbed his tallit (prayer shawl), and flushed it down the toilet. This was relayed to me, as with nearly all of Sam's "adventures," with thinly suppressed eruptions of laughter while turning red in an effort to constrain himself. Through this early memory I discerned that the very idea or mention of the word "toilet" would stimulate uncontrollable laughter in Sam.

Our early sessions were largely devoted to Sam's daily difficulties with his father at work, particularly in any area where his father behaved as his "boss." One such area of contention arose whenever Sam was commanded to clean the toilet in the shop. Sam would invariably reply, "What am I, the Mexican?" – a racial slur, one among many, that he uttered as a protest against what he felt was labor beneath him. Although Sam would then clean the toilet, this would always elicit an outburst of teasing, always at his father's expense. Consequently his father "fired" him many times, only to immediately hire him back.

Further into the treatment, after I confronted him on his frequent racist remarks, Sam relayed a story from childhood that again featured toilets. He described how his parents placed him in a more affordable public school near his hometown, one that he characterized as socially tough. As one of the only white students in the school who was, in addition, morbidly obese, he was constantly teased. This reached its most intense climax whenever he went to the bathroom. There, he reported, the black students would routinely put his head in the toilet. It is unclear what else transpired as he would not reveal more than this to me. And while he claimed to still hold residual rage against black males for this treatment, he again laughed in such a way as if to indicate an unexpected, and somewhat inappropriate pleasure from the way he was treated. As though he too found it funny when he imagined the experience through the eyes of those treating him sadistically, as though in some way he may have participated in his own mistreatment. The combined impact of his recollection and presentation of these events suggested to me that they were even now, in the telling, exciting if not arousing. In my experience, his presentation was not dissimilar to a report of a sexual fantasy. This reversal of expected affect, and suggestion of pleasure at his own debasement in a toilet, led me to consider Sam's experience in the psychoanalytic context of anal erotism.

Beginning with Freud as a starting point, there is a long history of efforts to theorize the psychological significance of the scatological and the abject in human life. According to Freudian theory, under ordinary circumstances the anus becomes a highly cathected (charged) erogenous zone during the psychosexual "anal" stage that is linked with toilet training.

> Praise and the fear of punishment play a powerful role in the domestication of the excretory sphincter ... Aggressive manifestations break out with vigor and are usually met by an environment equally determined to control them. The child's impulsive aggressive behavior (biting, hitting, pushing) becomes subject to repression ....
>
> Blos (1967, 20)

For a psychoanalyst, the significance of this chapter in any individual's life, especially Sam's life, cannot be overestimated. Freud (1957a, 187) notes,

> ... the first prohibition which a child comes across – the prohibition against getting pleasure from the anal activity and its products – has a decisive effect on his whole development. This must be the first occasion

on which the infant has a glimpse of an environment hostile to his instinctual impulses, on which he learns to separate his own entity from this alien one and on which he carries out the first 'repression' of his possibilities for pleasure. From that time on, what is 'anal' remains the symbol of everything that is to be repudiated and excluded from life.

So important is the outcome of this struggle between the infant's body and his/her environment that Freud (1961, 96–97) would posit that the rise of civilization itself rested on the successful repression of the aggressive strivings associated with the anal stage:

[Regarding] the anal erotism of young human beings ... Their original interest in the excretory function, its organs and products, is changed in the course of their growth into a group of traits which are familiar to us as parsimony, a sense of order and cleanliness – qualities which, though valuable and welcome in themselves, may be intensified till they become markedly dominant and produce what is called the anal character. How this happens we do not know, but there is no doubt about the correctness of the finding. Now we have seen that order and cleanliness are important requirements of civilization, although their vital necessity is not very apparent.

The incitement to cleanliness originates in an urge to get rid of the excreta, which have become disagreeable to sense perceptions. We know that in the nursery things are different. The excreta arouse no disgust in children. They seem valuable to them as being a part of their own body which has come away from it. Here upbringing insists with special energy on hastening the course of development which lies ahead, and which should make the excreta worthless, disgusting, abhorrent, and abominable. Such a reversal of values would scarcely be possible if the substances that are expelled from the body were not doomed by their strong smells to share the fate which overtook olfactory stimuli after man adopted the erect posture. Anal erotism, therefore, succumbs in the first instance to the 'organic repression' which paved the way to civilization.

100

Corresponding to the new dominance of repression in the life of the human child is the emergence of aggression. Specifically regarding anal aggression, Heimann (1989, 172) elaborates,

The first anal sub-stage is characterized by the aim of expulsion, and expresses the wish to annihilate the subject, whereas in the second anal sub-stage with the aim of retention a change in object relationships appears as the wish to preserve the object on condition that it be totally under the subject's control.

Freud (1959, 169) had already described the social appearance of anal repression in the character traits of those who are "orderly, parsimonious, and obstinate." Of particular importance,

> it is during the anal phase that the component instincts of sadism and masochism make their first and unmistakable appearance. In the helpless rage characteristic of the tantrum, both components are short-circuited: soon, however, *they find innumerable displacements of object and aim.*
>
> Blos (1967, 20, emphasis added)

Sam's wish for a cathartic, anally informed release through our treatment was initially displaced and symbolically expressed through prank phone calls scheduling home visits to his adversaries, real or imagined, from the plumbing company Roto-Rooter. Roto-Rooter was publicly associated with unclogging pipes. Their well-known television advertisement jingle was, "Call Roto-Rooter, that's the name, and away go troubles down the drain."

As a recurring subject of our sessions, Sam's comments on toilets are captured in this typical vignette which transpired after I questioned him on the Roto-Rooter prank:

> I don't know why I do it. I just get restless. I can't explain it. I'm not mad at anybody. I just have to do it when I get bored. I get bored and I need to shake things up a little. I just think these things are funny, don't you [smiling]?
>
> I don't understand why people get upset when I tell them about these things. I can't tell you why, I just find these things funny [laughing].
>
> It's like toilets, I can't stop laughing whenever I think about them.
>
> I need help with that because it might get me into trouble; like, what if I'm out on a date and my date says she has to go to the toilet, and I can't stop laughing. What do I do then?
>
> In all the time I've known you, you haven't been able to stop me from laughing.

Thus far my interpretation of Sam's past and present erotic behavior hinged on the notion of failed repression, of both his aggressive/sadistic impulses as well as the sexual delight he took in enacting them. Ferenczi (1980a, 180) writes, in support of my understanding: "Laughter is a failure of repression. A defense symptom against unconscious pleasure."

At the risk of replicating the original toilet-training struggle in the treatment, I felt with Sam, more than I usually do, an imperative need to establish an explicit frame or structure for his treatment right from the outset. This pertained to all features of our treatment "contract": the fee, time of our appointment, length of session, therapist neutrality, and so on. Langs (1977, 39–40) provides a clear rationale for this:

> The analyst should constantly monitor the state of the framework and each of its components: its holding functions, its containing functions, its role in creating a distinctive boundary for the analytic situation, and contributions to the therapeutic qualities of the field. Technically, this implies quiet attention to the various ground rules and boundaries, including an assessment of his own interventions in order to determine whether they have in any way modified his anonymity, neutrality, or attitude of not gratifying the patient's or his own inappropriate wishes.

I further modified my implementation of Lang's aforementioned frame to emphasize what Winnicott (1991) referred to as the "holding environment." Winnicott formulated the holding stage to address mothers responding to their infants for whom "being and annihilation are the two alternatives. The holding environment therefore has as its main function the reduction to a minimum of impingements to which the infant must react with resultant annihilation of personal being" (47). Given Sam's level of psychological functioning, his unwillingness to engage out of curiosity, and his repudiation of insight, I could not assume his ability to use me as an auxiliary ego, an analytic model, or an object to identify with (see Winnicott 1980 for a discussion of the fundamental importance of how objects may be used in treatment). Rather, Sam's disinclination toward insight betrayed a style of relating that appeared fully experiential, unconscious, and unmediated by self-awareness. Consequently, I adjusted myself to a style of relating that did not presume object differentiation (an even more primitive version of the Freudian anal stage, for that matter). I came to understand Sam's style of relating as *projective identification* in line with the object-relations theory of psychoanalysis.

"In projective identification parts of the [patient's] self and internal objects are split off and projected into the external object [therapist], which then becomes possessed by, controlled and identified with the projected parts" (Segal 1974, 27). The technical management of projective identification in treatment is clearly described by Ogden (1979) and was very pertinent to my work with Sam:

> The fantasy of putting a part of oneself into another person and controlling them from within reflects a central aspect of projective identification ... The projector feels that the recipient experiences his feeling, not merely a feeling like his own, but his own feeling that has been transplanted into the recipient ... one feels profoundly connected with the object ... (358); To summarize, projective identification is a set of

fantasies and object relations that can be schematically conceptualized as occurring in three phases: first, the fantasy of ridding oneself of an unwanted part of oneself and of putting that part into another person in an unwanted way; then the induction of feelings in the recipient that are congruent with the projective fantasy by means of an interpersonal interaction; and finally, the processing of the projection by the recipient, followed by the re-internalization by the projector of the 'metabolized projection.'

362

How might this process look with Sam? When he presented an episode to me that involved an impulsive/sadistic/expulsive act at someone else's expense and then giggled, waiting for me to join his laughter and sadistic delight, I would metabolize the form and content of his presentation as it transpired internally for me in a manner something like this: he is laughing (I don't know why); he is laughing somewhat ashamedly (something bad or wrong seems to have happened, uh-oh); he is signaling that he can't control himself (I'm not sure I can control him or what's he's done); he is taking delight in his own failure to control himself (he is in control of how chaotic this all is and he's manipulating it on purpose which is threatening); another person (or people) as described in his narrative was hurt (he might be dangerous or, worse, evil); he is scared (I am scared). My metabolized response, offered verbally for his reincorporation (imagine a bird chewing food to feed to its newborn offspring), would be to observe how anxious and intense the experience seems for him (and me), thereby converting my affective experience of him into concrete, articulable words. In this example I am the container, the holding environment, the auxiliary ego helping him digest his own seemingly uncontrollable affects. The telos of a treatment that inches forward in this way is based on a process that Kohut (1969) famously referred to as "transmuting internalization" – a belief that Sam will gradually, through a primitive identification process, adopt and assimilate my patient, analytical, self-regulatory ability.

Ultimately, the unstated goal of treatment was to enable Sam to sublimate, to self-regulate, to hold it together. But whose unarticulated, unagreed-on goal was this: Sam's, his parents', society's, or mine? The theoretical edifice on which my goal was based began with a certain understanding of wasting as vacating, or as a morally sanctioned evacuation of taboo (excremental) objects. Freud's emphasis on the formative influence of toilet training assumes a society pitted against a toddler with the singular goal of repression, for the sake of civilization no less. That which is repressed is the child's fascination with their own excrement – a fascination which precedes the taboo on these excreted objects that for the child are not necessarily differentiated from self, much less deemed impure – *the excreta arouse no disgust in children*. Following this line of the child's early relationship to their excremental processes, anal discharge may have been initially experienced as a prototypical release, not only from internal gastrointestinal discomfort but additionally from the surplus beyond the carrying capacity of what is functionally required to survive.

As Stoekl (2007, 36) notes,

> living organisms always, eventually, produce more than they need for simple survival and reproduction. Up to a certain point, their excess energy is channeled into expansion ... but inevitably the expansion of a species comes against limits: pressure will be exerted against insurmountable barriers.

Regarding these limits, Bataille (1991j, 30, emphases added) states,

> life suffocates within limits that are too close; it aspires in manifold ways to an impossible growth; it *releases a steady flow of excess resources,* possibly involving large squanderings of energy. The limits of growth being reached, life, without being in a closed container, at least enters into *ebullition.* Without exploding, *its extreme exuberance pours out* in a movement always bordering on *an explosion.*

According to Bataille, these "limits of growth" are manifest in the taboo systems general to our society, including toilet training, and this inevitable "pouring out" takes on the form of the taboo's transgression: "There exists no prohibition that cannot be transgressed. Often the transgression is permitted, often it is even prescribed" (Bataille 1986b, 63).

This alternate line of inquiry in empathy with the child's early excremental experience emphasizes not repression and regulation but rather "the refusal to limit the self [and] our desire to fuse, to mingle, to blend [which] requires a partial dissolution of self" (Cullen 1997, 14). Again, Canetti (1993, 17, author's emphasis), affirms the same process writ large within the social body:

> The most important occurrence within the crowd is the *discharge.* Before this the crowd does not actually exist; it is the discharge which creates it. This is the moment when all who belong to the crowd get rid of their differences and feel equal.

Bataille (1991e, 67) himself consistently emphasizes "the necessity of throwing oneself out of oneself." This represents a shift from an emphasis on repression and containment (along with the accumulation-through-internalization model of mental health that this implies) to an unbounded, undifferentiated, ecstatic experience of self-in-environment.

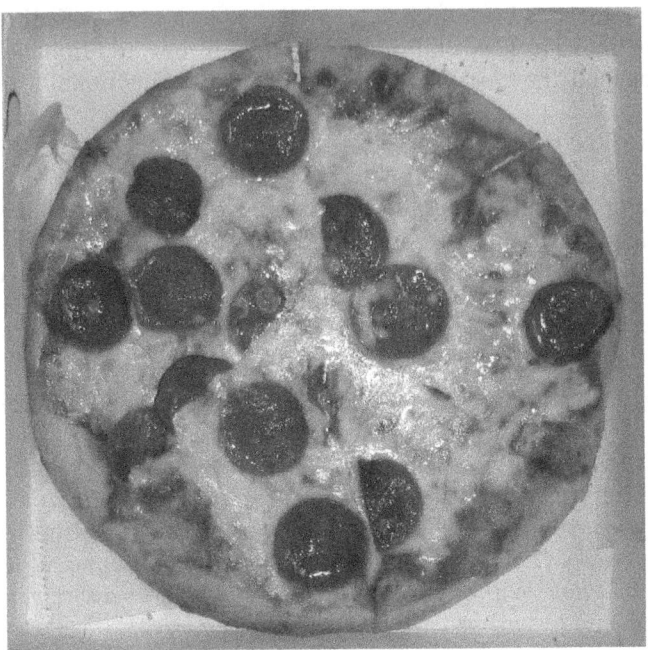

Figure 5.2 Pizza.

From the very beginning of his treatment, Sam developed a ritual of pizza-binging on his way to see me. His workplace was located across town from my office. Due to his work hours I agreed to see him in the late afternoon. He informed me almost immediately that he would use our appointments as an excuse to leave work early; he would make several, intermittent stops at pizza parlors walking on his way to my office, ordering a slice here and there, ultimately consuming the equivalent of an entire large pizza pie en route to our session. Most times this resulted in him falling asleep while sitting up during the session in a post-binge daze. I would be reduced to a silent witness, sitting and gazing at a man entirely given over to his internal process of digestion.

In that "consumption is destruction to the extent that it is loss or waste" (Kendall 2019, 90), I experienced Sam's blatant exhibition of his digestive process after excess consumption as aggressive. It begged the imperative question of when and how he would evacuate – the implied metaphorical, corporeal *modus operandi* of Sam's treatment goal. He seemed to mock my ideas of containing and holding by reducing me to therapist-as-toilet, waiting for the excremental bits that could not be digested. Nietzsche captured this moment exactly, if not ironically:

We all live this way! We greedily devour things with our insatiable eyes, and then just as greedily empty them of whatever flatters our task or might be useful to us – and then leave the bits our teeth and our appetite could not finish off to others and to nature, especially the bits we could not digest: our excrement. This means we are not greedy at all, we are inexhaustibly generous: we bestow on humanity's *dungpile* what our spirit and our experiences found indigestible.

   Nietzsche quoted in Blondel (1991, 222, author's emphasis)

Pragmatically speaking, after overeating Sam was unavailable to "take in" anything I said or did that might affect him. It is though Sam grasped, at least physically, that the entire therapy process was one of digestion and that, in the same sense that I might take him in and metabolize our experience for him, he might in turn eventually be expected to reincorporate me (see Meissner 1981 on the crucial distinction between the primal process of incorporation as distinct from introjection and identification within the developmental spectrum of internalization possibilities). In that respect, Sam's zoning out in front of me might be psychoanalytically construed as a primitive defense mechanism, one of the "pathological states of deep, so-called narcissistic regression" (Jacobson 1964, 9). Moreover, to the extent that psychological trauma itself may be understood through the metaphor of digestion, Sam's alimentary defense against engaging verbally and articulating his experience suggested to me a concrete reenactment of early trauma. My conjecture was based on an etiological notion of trauma as an early confrontation with an experience or object too large to break down by an immature psychological digestive system. (Winnicott (1974) notes that the mental breakdown most feared is one already experienced but inadequately digested at a tender, earlier, and undeveloped time in life.)

   Phenomenologically speaking, Sam's therapy ritual of excessive intake and mindless digestion appeared to be a parody of the treatment. In this view, the labor of his digestive processes concretely mimed the labor of therapy, requiring as it does the internalization of therapeutic insight and experience. If, as Strachey (1934) claimed, the psychological "mutative" transformation sought in therapy occurs when the patient is confronted with an interpersonal reality contra his/her transferential or fantasied expectations, what was Scott communicating to me?

   The sheer excess of food Sam consumed, as well as his excessive body size, created a concrete symbol of disproportion that privileged Sam's body over his mind, thus dis-privileging insight, theorizing, and the *a priori* bias of therapy toward cerebral interiority. Contrary to a psychosexual interpretation invoking oral motivations or early anal trauma to express the function and telos of excessive consumption, Sam's eating also alternatively "represents appropriation as a means of excretion" (Bataille 1991g, 99) and thus a reversal from the usual emphasis on interpreted meaning to a strange highlighting of useless discharge. Bataille (1991g, 99), captured my frustration, disgust, and ultimate wish to laugh in the throes of this alternative, embodied perspective on therapy:

> as soon as the effort at rational comprehension ends in contradiction, the practice of intellectual scatology requires the excretion of unassimilable elements, which is another way of stating vulgarly that a burst of laughter is the only imaginable and definitively terminal result – not the means – of philosophical speculation.

As I proceeded to explore the subject of pizzas, I noticed that, as with the subject of toilets, pizzas also precipitated the twinkling eyes, blushing, and eruptions of laughter from Sam. I came to learn that for sport, for revenge, or just for a laugh, Sam would have pizzas delivered to people within his neighborhood or near his job. The titillation and glee he experienced were due to both the shock and dismay of the recipient as well as the costly, distressing impact on the delivery person and pizza parlor involved. Our discussion of this behavior, rather than mollifying it by subjecting it to the secondary, regulatory process of verbal narrative, actually intensified it. Sam seemed to mistake my interest in these "deliveries" as my sanctioning them. His trust in me developed to the extent that I was viewed as a co-conspirator or accomplice who, again, was "in on the joke." He described, in great detail, how he regularly increased the intensity of the delivery excitement by ordering several pizza pies with all the toppings to inculcate greater and greater outrage within those affected.

He was not remorseful in the least, nor do I believe he was afraid of being caught. In fact, I think his full fantasy of the delivery event would culminate in a final, violent exposure and confrontation with painfully humiliating consequences for him. Moreover, as with the boys who debased him in the stalls of his high school bathrooms, he seemed to be aroused by this nearly intolerable but seemingly desired outcome. Bataille (1991g, 101), again, provides comment directly related to this form of Sam's pleasure:

> it is true that one of man's attributes is the derivation of pleasure from the suffering of others, and that erotic pleasure is not only the negation of an agony that takes place at the same instant, but also a lubricious participation in that agony.

The functional importance of the mouth for human subsistence and survival is obvious. Less obviously, the mouth is identified as the physical foundation and model for the psychological process of incorporation and a crucial metaphor for understanding how Sam formed and related to his world.

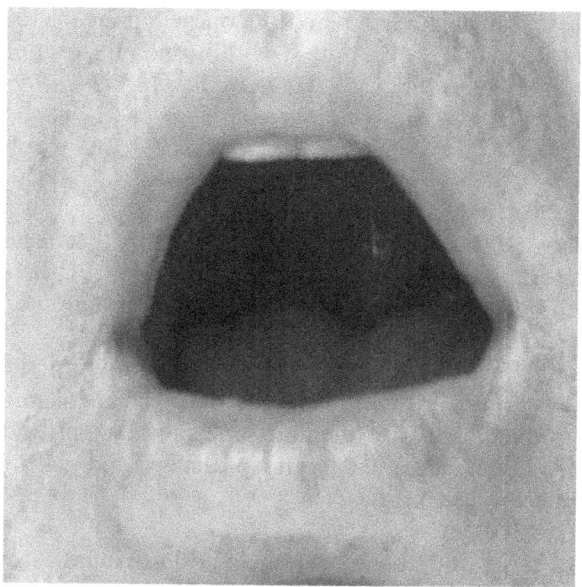

Figure 5.3 Mouth.

According to the American Psychiatric Association (1975, 90, author's emphases): incorporation is "a primitive *defense mechanism*, operating *unconsciously*, in which the psychic representation of a person or parts of him, are figuratively ingested." Klein (1977, 291) provides a more elaborate, if not arcane, psychoanalytic take on this psychiatric notion of incorporation:

> By this is meant the mental activity in the child, by which, in his fantasy, he takes into himself everything which he perceives in the outside world. We know that at this stage the child receives his main satisfaction through his mouth, which therefore becomes the main channel through which the child takes in not only his food, but also, in his fantasy, the world around him.

Jacobson (1964) further expands Klein's definition of incorporation, by accentuating the concomitant loss of individuation and differentiation between self and object; and Meissner (1981) explicitly describes incorporation as the complete assimilation of the other in self.

The classic Freudian viewpoint on incorporation is provided by LaPlanche & Pontalis (1973) and, importantly, extends the potential malleability of the self-other distinction to an exchange, through displacement, between body parts and body functions:

Actually incorporation contains three meanings: it means to obtain pleasure by making an object penetrate oneself; it means to destroy this object; and it means, by keeping it within oneself, to appropriate the object's qualities ... *Similarly, there is an anal incorporation in so far as the rectal cavity is identified with the mouth.*

212 (emphasis added)

In a Freudian sense, displacement up, from anus to mouth, is accentuated and reinforced by the identical potential for discharge between both. "The mouth and the anus bear an undeniable connection. They are literally connected, each being one end of a tube that runs through the body ... the one often represents the other" (Miller 1997, 96).

For Bataille, the reversal of emphasis between bodily functions becomes complete as the mouth is the site of not only the incorporative act of devouring but, linked as it is to the anus, the site of eruptive discharge as well – through laughter, screams, vomit, spittle, and so on. To wit, Bataille (1991d, 59, emphasis added) states,

It is easy to observe that the overwhelmed individual throws back his head while frenetically stretching his neck in such a way that the mouth becomes, as much as possible, an extension of the spinal column, in other words, in the position it normally occupies in the constitution of animals. As if explosive impulses were to spurt directly out of the body through the mouth, in the form of screams. This fact highlights both the importance of the mouth in animal physiology or even psychology, *and the general importance of the superior or anterior extremity of the body, the orifice of profound physical impulses.*

Bataille's focus on the notion of laughter-as-discharge has a precedent in medieval carnival. As described by Bakhtin (1984), laughter/discharge fulfills not only a biological but a social release as well. As a political levelling effect, it offers a critical response to any and all hierarchical structures. As such, several aspects of Bakhtin's discussion are illuminating with regard to Sam's position vis-à-vis his father. Regarding "carnival laughter," Bakhtin (1984) notes,

it is not an individual reaction to some isolated 'comic' event. Carnival laughter is the laughter of all the people. Second, it is universal in scope; it is directed at all and everyone, including the carnival's participants. The entire world is seen in its droll aspect, in its gay relativity. Third, this laughter is ambivalent: it is gay, triumphant, and at the same time mocking, deriding. It asserts and denies, it buries and revives ... it is also directed at those who laugh.

11–12

As with the carnival participant, Sam's laughter ultimately, either directly or indirectly, implicated himself. Like any trickster, he always ended up the butt of his own jokes: "The depressive disposition of most clowns seems to indicate that the attempt to tear down the envied rival, who unconsciously stands for the father, does not remain unpunished" (Reich 1973, 116). But also like any trickster, Sam's experiences of defilement additionally offered release and renewal.

> Carnival laughter, then, has a vulgar, 'earthy' quality to it. With its oaths and profanities, its abusive language and its mocking words it was profoundly ambivalent. Whilst it humiliated and mortified it also revived and renewed ... ritual defilements went along with reinvigoration.
>
> Stallybrass and White (1992, 8)

The ambivalence of laughter in connection to the carnival pertained to the theatricality of Sam's world as regularly enacted by him:

> 'Destructive humor' is not directed against isolated negative aspects of reality but against all reality, against the finite world as a whole. All that is finite is per se destroyed by humor ... Through it, the entire world is turned into something alien, something terrifying and unjustified. The ground slips from under our feet, and we are terrified because we find nothing stable around us ... All that was frightening in ordinary life is turned into amusing or ludicrous monstrosities.
>
> Bakhtein (1984, 42–47)

What does a shift in emphasis to laughter-as-discharge mean for treatment? In Bataille's "general economy" terms, the mouth is restored to its full ambivalent importance in life: Introjection as devouring equals production; laughter as discharge equals wasteful expenditure, or, as noted earlier, an urge to purge, to evacuate – not only excrement, pizzas, words, hierarchical structures, or reality but meaning itself. Bataille (1986a, 90) elaborates,

> Let us suppose that that which induces laughter is not only unknown, but unknowable. There is still one possibility to be considered. That which is laughable may simply be the unknowable. In other words, the unknown nature of the laughable would be not accidental, but essential. We would laugh, not for some reason which, due to a lack of information, or of sufficient penetration, we shall never manage to know, but because the unknown makes us laugh. We laugh, in short, in passing very abruptly, all of a sudden, from a world in which everything is firmly qualified, in which everything is given as stable within a generally stable order, into a world in which our assurance is overwhelmed, in which we perceive that this assurance was deceptive. Where everything had

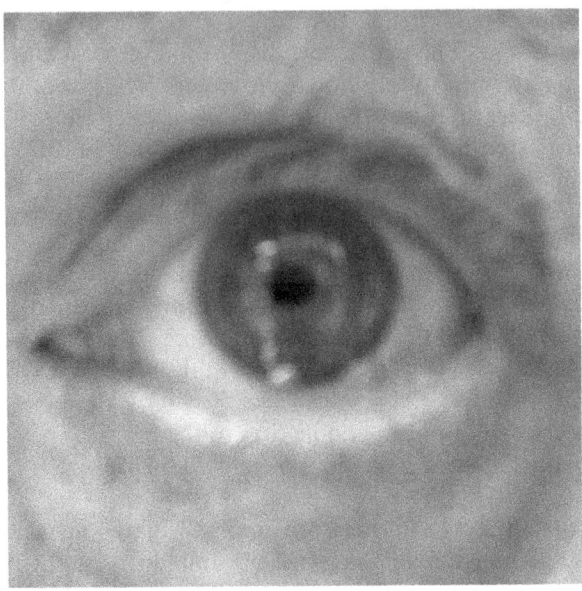

Figure 5.4 Eye.

seemed totally provided for, suddenly the unexpected arises, something unforeseeable and overwhelming, revelatory of an ultimate truth: the surface of appearances conceals a perfect absence of response to our expectation.

Sam needed to be present for all his pranks. Only by visually witnessing an episode could he take full credit for it, that is, ratify it as real and separate from his fantasy life in order to achieve full gratification. Moreover, it was a bonus beyond measure if the aggrieved or flummoxed victims of his pranks saw him watching. This level of non-verbal interaction served as a visual corollary to the aforementioned projective-identification. To begin with, "the act of directly looking is the equivalent of identification" (Bataille 1991f, 74). In its more primitive manifestation of identification, the eye itself incorporates.

Fenichel (1953, 373–374) elaborates on the psychoanalytic perspective that "to look = to devour" and that "the idea of devouring … represents a form of sadistic incorporation." In other words, "'I wish what I see to enter into me'" (378), and by this means, "the person looking makes an onslaught with his eye upon the world, in order to 'devour' it" (379) through a process of "ocular introjection" (389).

Fenichel, further expands on the sexual aspect of visuality in his discussion of scopophilia – "the sexual pleasure in looking" – and notes that "when subserving the scopophilic instinct, the eye is to be regarded as an erotogenic zone" (376). This builds on Freud's (1957b, 216–218) analysis of scopophilia in which he asserts "that an organ normally serving the purpose of sense-perception begins to behave like an actual genital when its erotogenic role is increased." Thus Fenichel (1953, 389) asserts the potential for an experience of "the eye as a phallic symbol," a relationship further affirmed in folklore by Griaule (1995) and through surrealist art by Krauss (1993).

Freud (1957a, 192) explores the etiology of scopophilia and connects it with early excretion: "Since opportunities for satisfying curiosity of this kind usually occur only in the course of satisfying the two kinds of need for excretion, children of this kind turn into voyeurs, eager spectators of the processes of micturition and defecation." Fenichel (1953, 377, author's emphases) affirming Freud, goes on to conjecture a combination of visuality, identification, and destruction within the watching-excreting relationship:

> the aim of the scopophilic instinct is *to look at* the sexual object ... to watch him or her performing the functions of excretion ... one looks at an object *to share in* its experience ... Very often sadistic impulses enter into the instinctual aim of looking: one wishes *to destroy* something by means of looking at it, or else the act of looking itself has already acquired the significance of a modified form of destruction.

For Bataille (1991b, 17) the eye is classically, ostensibly the ideal purveyor of truth through which the "fear of the eye" is related to "the *eye of conscience*." However, the eye is not neutral, "The relationship between viewer and scene is always one of fracture, partial identification, pleasure, and distrust" (Rose 1996, 227). In fact, "... the eye itself could have several conflicting meanings for Bataille" (Jay 1994, 22) that extend well beyond the eye of conscience; as when "the eye is toppled from its privileged place in the sensual hierarchy to be linked instead with objects and functions more normally associated with 'baser' human behavior" (221), and there in a debased, profaned state is where Sam lives, while "his eyes continue to fetter him tightly to vulgar things" (Bataille 1991i, 83).

Sam was visually aroused through his identification with the injury of the wronged party as well as the possibility of his being seen – all given away by his laughter and blushing. Even his blushing was implicated in the scopophilic act: "The blushing of our patient thus says, 'See my erection (defecation), be excited with me'" (Schilder 1978, 239). For Sam, the eyes were portals to an un-mediated sadistic experience that he visually devoured, like pizza – the sexual excitement of each episode being dangerously excessive. That is, if he stared too long, he would be overexposed.

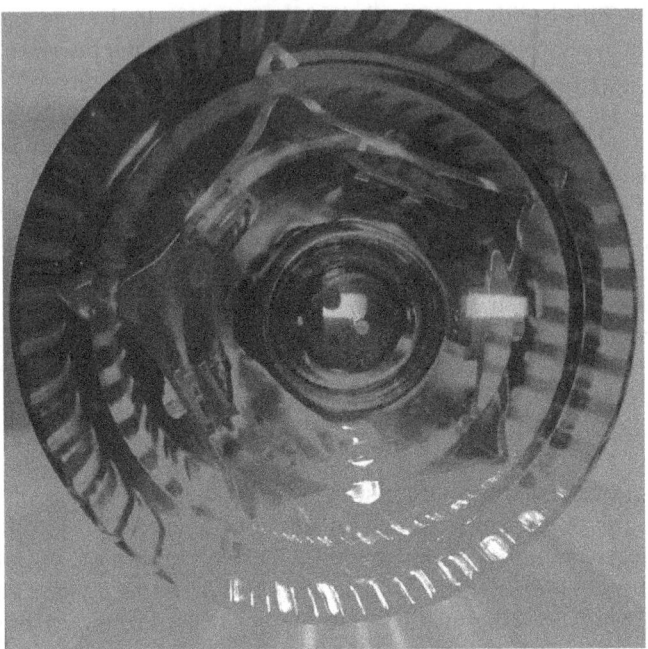

Figure 5.5 Emergency.

When Sam tired of pizza pranks he moved onto larger and costlier deliveries, for example Dial-a-Mattress. On a dare, he fell asleep undressed on the back of a fire truck during a short stint as a volunteer fireman. When the firetruck pulled out in response to an emergency, he was publicly exposed and humiliated. This prank, along with his abrupt dismissal from the fire department, fueled his friends' and his own amusement and laughter. Still, Scott's "boredom" and restlessness always returned and finally culminated in his most outrageous act.

One afternoon I was sitting in a session listening to the patient that preceded Sam when there came a knock on my door. It was too early for Sam's usual arrival time so I went outside to inquire. A police officer greeted me in the waiting room. Sam was standing next to him. He asked me if I knew Sam which I affirmed. The officer proceeded to relate an episode that had just transpired outside my door. He said that Sam was sitting in his car parked right in front of my building when he decided to call 911, the New York City emergency number, and told the operator that a police officer had been shot and "was down" in the building directly across the street from mine. The officer, in an agitated and threatening tone told me that Sam was "very sick" and that I better "straighten him out." The officer left, leaving Sam in my waiting room, in my care. When I later commenced the session with Sam as scheduled, he informed me that he did in fact make the call. He said he wanted to watch all the police cars converge right in front of him outside his car window. Scott described how, in the midst of the chaos that ensued on the street, one of the police officers calmly walked over and knocked on the passenger window of his car. Sam opened the window and the officer asked if he could get in. Once inside, the officer asked him why he did it. Sam answered in what I believe was a shocked and sheepish but sincere manner, "I have a generalized anxiety disorder." The officer responded, "What the fuck is a generalized anxiety disorder?" At that point, Sam invoked my name pointing at my building and said he was waiting for his appointment with me. As Sam reported the details of the event, he was not laughing but actually seemed relieved, as though he finally found a way to calm himself down.

I tried to take advantage of the relative calm in our sessions following the police incident. We explored the more vulnerable side of his feelings related to his adoption. I was following a hunch that, given Sam's daily acrimonious exchanges with his father, while his mother passively observed, he may not feel that he belonged in his adoptive family nor that his parents, crucially, "love him for his own sake and as a person in his own right" (Guntrip 1961, 284). With some encouragement from me Sam went to check the city birth registry

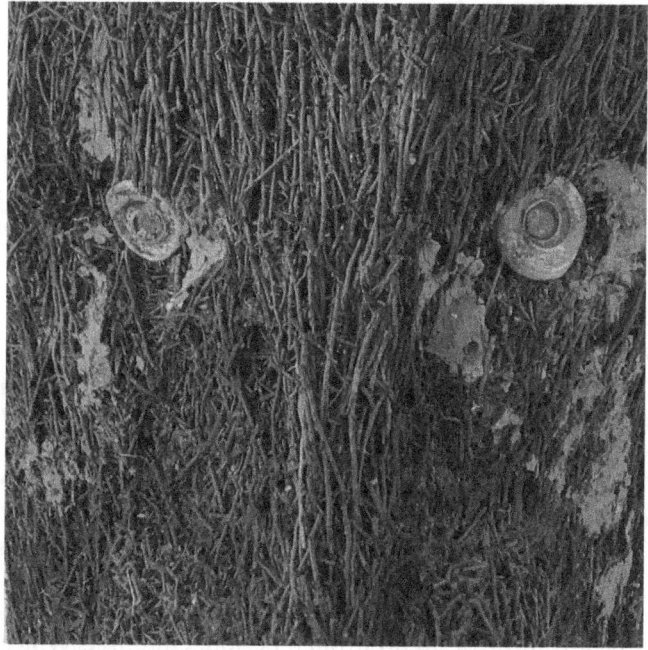

Figure 5.6 Excremental man.

in an effort to locate his biological family of origin and the cause of his abandonment. One day, after Cancelling a series of sessions, he sat with me and reported that he had some information. While he could not locate the names of his parents, he was able to locate his place of birth. He sheepishly told me that he was born in Mexico City and then burst into uncontrollable laughter. I knew he was laughing at himself and I also knew he was not open to taking in anything that I would say in that moment. Then he got up and left.

That evening, following Sam's revelation, I stopped to use my bathroom before leaving. When I flushed the toilet the water came surging out, uncontrollably, flooding my floor. After I shut off the main water line, I looked inside the tank to find it had been vandalized.

As a way of trying to cope with this destructive act aimed at me, I tried to name it (if not understand it). I immediately (and defensively) sought to manage my feelings by objectifying Sam and invoking the appropriate behaviorally oriented psychiatric diagnosis, thus extricating myself from him, our relationship, and our process. I reasoned that Scott was suffering from an Intermittent Explosive Disorder (DSM V, #312.34) (American Psychiatric Association 2013, 466–467, emphasis added), formally defined as:

A Recurrent behavioral outbursts representing a failure to control aggressive impulses as manifested by either of the following:
   1 Verbal aggression (e.g., temper tantrums, tirades, verbal arguments, or fights) or physical aggression toward property, animals, or other individuals, occurring twice weekly, on average, for a period of three months. The physical aggression does not result in damage or destruction of property and does not result in physical injury to animals or other individuals.
   2 Three behavioral outbursts involving damage or destruction of property and/or physical assault involving physical injury against animals or other individuals occurring within a 12-month period of time.
B *The magnitude of aggressiveness expressed during the recurrent outbursts is grossly out of proportion to the provocation or to any precipitating psychosocial stressor.*
C The recurrent aggressive outbursts are not premeditated (i.e., they are impulsive and/or anger-based) and *are not committed to achieve some tangible objective* (e.g., money, power, intimidation)
D The recurrent aggressive outbursts cause either marked distress in the individual or impairment in occupational or interpersonal functioning, or are associated with financial or legal consequences.
   Diagnostic Features: The impulsive (or anger-based) aggressive outbursts in intermittent explosive disorder have a rapid onset and, typically, little or no prodromal period. Outbursts typically last for less than 30 minutes and commonly occur in response to a minor provocation by a close intimate or associate.

The explosion in my bathroom had revolted me and I felt overwhelmed from without and within. I remained angry at Sam until I saw him for our session the following week. When I confronted him right at the outset about the broken toilet, he repeatedly swore that he did not do it. However, his lies were betrayed by his twinkling, blushing, and, above all, his laughing – a laughter I viscerally felt was sadistically at my expense. My anger with him grew to a level I could not accept, much less contain or metabolize, and I terminated his treatment then and there.

With time and distance I struggled to recover a more neutral, process-oriented, psychoanalytically informed understanding of the event that resulted in my termination of Sam's treatment. Certainly it seemed to be what is typically referred to as "acting out" in the treatment – on both of our parts.

In its most neutral manifestation,

> The term *acting out* thus properly refers to any behavior that is assumed to be an expression of transference attitudes that the patient does not yet feel safe to bring into treatment in words ... What is acted out may be predominantly self-destructive, or predominantly growth-enhancing, or some of each; what makes it acting out is not its goodness or badness but the unconscious and fearsome nature of the impulses that propel the person into action and the compulsive automatic way in which the acting-out behavior in undertaken.
>
> McWilliams (1994, 139)

This general definition focuses, like the psychiatric DSM diagnosis provided above, on the behavioral quality of the acting out, that is, the impulsivity. However, more particularly relevant to my treatment of Sam was the relationship between repression, aggression, and discharge. Acting out,

> is action in which the subject, in the grip of unconscious wishes and phantasies, relives these in the present with a sensation of immediacy which is heightened by his refusal to recognize their source and their repetitive character ... Such action generally displays an impulsive aspect relatively out of harmony with the subject's usual motivational patterns ... Acting out often takes the form of aggressive behavior directed either at the self or at others.
>
> LaPlanche and Pontalis (1973, 4)

"the act is ill-motivated even in the subject's own eyes, constituting a radical departure from his usual behavior even if he rationalizes it after the fact. For the psychoanalyst indications such as these betoken the *return of the repressed*" (5, author's emphasis). To this Freudian take on acting out, Fenichel adds the importance of the transferential reenactment of the drama with the parents:

The impulses of the patient have once before met with prohibitions, which was the cause of his pathogenic repressions. An analyst who actively prohibits his patient's impulses might be perceived as a replica of the parents, who once forbade the utterances of infantile [anal] sexuality.

Fenichel (1954, 303)

all neurotic acting out has the following in common: It is an acting which unconsciously relieves inner tension and brings a partial discharge to warded-off impulses … the present situation, somehow associatively connected with the repressed content, is used as an occasion for the discharge of repressed energies.

296

As compelling and plausible as the above psychoanalytic formulations are, all the classical or psychiatric definitions of acting out still seemed incomplete. I required more than a generic rationalization of his behavior, I needed to understand Sam in the context of our specific story. The first glimpse of a way forward in my drama with Sam came from Bataille scholar Kendall (2019) who states,

Whether the waste derives from our own bodies or behaviors, or from outside of us in the workings of the world, we struggle to recast it, to interpret, explain or otherwise tame its virulence, while nevertheless allowing ourselves, wittingly or unwittingly, consciously or unconsciously, to be caught up in its mechanisms.

89

Not only did this help me understand how I got "caught up," but Kendall's formulation helped me view "acting out" differently – as an inevitable waste product of any treatment. I was beginning to accord the notion of waste and wasting its proper place in my work. It took a very long time for me to accept emotionally, not just intellectually, "that there are lives not sustained by *desire*, as desire is always for objects. Such lives are based on *exclusion* … articulated by *negation* and its modalities, *transgression*, *denial*, and *repudiation* [and] dependent upon a dialectic of negativity" (Kristeva 1982, 6–7, author's emphasis).

The facts of our treatment, along with my understanding of Sam's history, seemed to indicate that he had successfully, once again, managed to recruit someone in order to have himself violently discharged or expelled. Moreover, it's altogether possible that our relationship was cultivated by Sam toward that aim. Was Sam's perpetual rejection his unconscious repetitive and compulsive enactment of his abandonment to adoption in infancy by his mother? If so, Sam would not accept the part of the injured victim forgotten and devalued by his mother or society. Rather, through a creative reversal of his life's narrative, Sam believed his social value lay in his identity as the excluded, extruded, vacated, and grotesque Other; as Homo Sacer – social outcast, yet still continuously punished (Agamben 1998). Stallbrass and White (1992, 191, author's emphases) describe a precedent for this peculiar social role in the figure of the "grotesque in" the Middle Ages:

> The bourgeois subject continuously defined and re-defined itself through the exclusion of what it marked out as 'low' – as dirty, repulsive, noisy, and contaminating. Yet that very act of exclusion, was constitutive of its identity. The low was internalized under the sign of negation and disgust.
>
> 191

> It nourished and replenished its refined formalisms from the symbolic repertoire of the grotesque body *in the very name of exclusion*. It took the grotesque within itself so as to reject it, but this meant only that the grotesque was now an unpalatable and interiorized *phobic* set of representations associated with avoidance and with others … It was always someone else who was possessed by the grotesque, never the self. In this way the bourgeois public sphere, that 'idealist' realm of judgement, refinement, wit and rationalism was dependent upon disavowal, denial, and projection.
>
> 108 (author's emphases)

By contrast with its social context,

> The grotesque body … has *its* discursive norms too: impurity (both in the sense of dirt and mixed categories), heterogeneity, masking, protuberant distension, disproportion, exorbitancy, clamor, decentered or eccentric arrangements, a focus on gaps, orifices and symbolic filth, physical needs and pleasures of the 'lower body stratum,' materiality and parody.
>
> 23 (author's emphasis)

Sam's active, repeated participation in his own exclusion, whether consciously or unconsciously, suggests strongly that he identified himself as excrement or as an excremental man. His primitive, erotic identification of himself as excrement, as that which is expelled, is not to be confused with the fetish of coprophilia, an "excessive or morbid interest in filth or feces or their symbolic representation" (APA 1975, 37), but as a complete, if not metaphorical, identification. The etiological factors contributing to how this identity is established is also the source of extensive psychoanalytic speculation.

By what path does excrement enter subjectification? ... The child is asked to hold it in. He is made to hold it in too long, to start to introduce excrement into the realm of what belongs to his body, which is considered, at least for a while, as something not to be lost.

Lacan (2018, 300–301)

Freud addresses the developmental precondition for this identification with excrement.

The contents of the bowels, which act as a stimulating mass upon a sexually sensitive portion of mucous membrane, behave like forerunners of another organ, which is destined to come into action after the phase of childhood. But they have other important meanings for the infant. They are clearly treated as a part of the infant's own body.

Freud (1957a, 186)

Additionally, Fleiss (1956, 134) refers to the aural derivative of this identification: "The spoken word under certain conditions is – as are feces in the anal phase – conceived of as part of the speaker (= speaker's body)."

As it turns out, Sam identified with the Mexican and Black individuals he so often derided. In his mind, they were also excremental people who were also routinely treated like shit. Extrapolated to an even larger political context, Sam's "acting out" behavior was analogous to a social cause, a revolution of sorts. Bataille (1991g, author's emphasis) describes,

Of course the term *excretion* applied to the Revolution must first be understood in the strictly mechanical – and moreover etymological – sense of the word. The first phase of the revolution is *separation*, in other words, a process leading to the position of two groups of forces, each one characterized by the necessity of excluding the other. The second phase is the violent *expulsion* of the group that has possessed power by the revolutionary group.

100

Moreover, in all instances of political suppression we observe that "The eruptive force accumulates in those who are necessarily situated below" (Bataille (1991a, 8). Again and again the notion of excrement or waste as dead matter, whether in the thought and actions of Sam or Bataille, shows itself to be something actually far less stable, even animate. "Such matter is in excess, not inert but virulent, threatening, turning as easily against the one who would wield the power as against a supposed victim" Stoekl (2007, 34). Consequently, the lives of the extruded or grotesque others will not sit easily in reified clinical, classificatory categories. "The leading themes of these images of bodily life are fertility, growth and a brimming-over abundance" (Stallbrass and White 1992, 9).

Figure 5.7 Sun.

Sam and I maintained contact in the years following my termination of his treatment. Through periodic phone calls he informed me that he had engaged in treatment again, was feeling better, and had taken a job as a security guard in a Manhattan museum. I felt, not thought, but bodily felt the irony of Sam spending his days ensuring the security of decomposing objects. He laughingly asked me if he could resume his therapeutic care with me and I declined. I sensed with Sam that his request wasn't about me or our connection as much as his need to hold onto the conviction that the repressed always can and will return. And that the ebullition of that return was still, even after all this time, synonymous with the erotic experience of self-destruction that Sam most desired.

> It would be inexcusable to speak of eroticism without saying essentially that it centers on joy. A joy, moreover, that is excessive ... there can be no doubt about the excessive, exorbitant character of the transports of joy that eroticism gives us ... Erotic activity can be disgusting; it can be noble, ethereal, excluding sexual contact, but it illustrates a principle of human behavior in the clearest way: what we want is what uses up our strength and our resources and, if necessary, places our life in danger ... the object we desire the most is in principle the one most likely to endanger or destroy us.
>
> Bataille (1991k, 103–104)

As a living paragon of expenditure, Sam exuded with all the ambivalence of the sun – always rising only to fall again; always eliciting my hope and expectations only to disappoint; always discharging, generating, radiating until it hurt himself and others; always laughing until the fun turned into fearful horror.

> The sun, from the human point of view (in other words, as it is confused with the notion of noon) is the most elevated concept. It is also the most abstract object, since it is impossible to look at it fixedly at that time of day … In practice the scrutinized sun can be identified with a mental ejaculation, foam on the lips, and an epileptic crisis. In the same way that the preceding sun (the one not looked at) is perfectly beautiful, the one that is scrutinized can be considered horribly ugly … All this leads one to say that the summit of elevation is in practice confused with a sudden fall of unheard-of violence … that which most ruptures the highest elevation, and for a blinding brilliance, has a share in the elaboration or decomposition of forms.
>
> Bataille (1991c, 57–58)

In our last phone conversation Sam let me know that his earlier ravaging of his body had caught up with him in the form of acute diabetes. He described what sounded like the gradual decomposition of his own body beginning with his extremities, that is, fingers and toes. In the past year, while writing this essay, I learned that Sam died at a relatively young age. He is biologically dead and yet I continue to metabolize him. He has been evacuated from the world but not from within me. All his amputated parts, his pranks, his stories, his shit, his gifts placed into me, they have all been lying inside for years, undigested … until now.

Thus, I present you with Sam in written form, as my own expulsion, as my own contribution to "the psycho-analytical dunghill, namely the analytic literature. A dunghill is a little pile of shit" (Lacan 2018, 302). After all, although this is Sam's story, "you can't imagine the cornucopia that can be assembled from the mere excrement of a mass of humanity" (300).

Moreover, I present Sam; convulsed, post-mortem, in photographic fragments. "As directed by the text that accompanies them, the photographs become interpretable as documents of convulsive beauty, objective and unconscious" (Ades 1985, 183).

> The word 'convulsive,' which I use to describe the only beauty which should concern us, would lose any meaning in my eyes were it to be conceived in motion and not at the exact expiration of this motion. There can be no beauty at all, as far as I'm concerned – convulsive beauty – except at the cost of affirming the reciprocal relations linking the object seen in its motion and in its repose.
>
> Breton (1988, 10)

the experience of something that has been in motion but has been, for some reason, stopped, derailed ... the convulsiveness, then, the arousal in front of the object is not to it perceived within the continuum of its natural existence, but detached from that flow by means of an expiration of motion, a detachment that deprives [it] of some part of its physical self and turns it into a sign of the reality it no longer possesses.

Krauss (1985, 31–32)

I offer you Sam, no longer the Sam who exploded through his days, his work, his family, and my office, but Sam finally stilled in death as a fixed-explosive:

> ... the fixed-explosive, nature arrested in motion ...The veiled-erotic, or reality convulsed into a writing, is a photographic effect, but fundamentally it concerns an uncanny trace of a prior state, i.e., of the compulsion to return to an ultimately inanimate condition [that is] The fixed-explosive, or reality convulsed in shock.

Foster (1993, 27–28)

It is in emulation of Sam that I offer this oblation for expiation as I hereby evict him, this solar annulus, "to which nothing sufficiently blinding can be compared except the sun, even though the anus is the *night*" (Bataille 1991a, 9, author's emphases).

Adieu, Sam. If all your treatments were a waste of time and energy, as your father and a series of psychotherapists would claim, should we not examine this waste to which your life was so adamantly devoted? Not only for

Figure 5.8 The spectral attraction of decomposition.

the scopophilic delight in it but as witnesses to a sacred act, as a sacrifice of yourself? A sacrifice so utterly excessive that we laugh until we cry?

> The sun, situated at the bottom of the sky like a cadaver at the bottom of a pit, answers this inhuman cry with the spectral attraction of decomposition ... fecal like the eye painted at the bottom of a vase, this Sun, now borrowing its brilliance from death, has buried existence in the stench of the night.
>
> Bataille (1991i, 84)

Bibliography

Abraham, Karl. "Contributions to the Theory of the Anal Character." In *Selected Papers on Psychoanalysis*, 370–392. Translated by Douglas Bryan and Alix Strachey. New York: Brunner/Mazel, 1927/1921.

Ades, Dawn. "Photography and the Surrealist Text." In *L'Amour Fou*, 155–194. Edited by Rosalind Krauss and Jane Livingston. New York: Abbeville Press, 1985.

Adler, Alfred. *The Individual Psychology of Alfred Adler: A Systematic Presentation in Selections from His Writings*. Edited by Heinz L. Ansbacher and Rowena R. Ansbacher. New York: Harper & Row, 1964.

Agamben, Giorgio. *Homo Sacer: Sovereign Power and Bare Life*. Translated by Daniel Heller-Roazen. Stanford, CA: Stanford University Press, 1998.

Aichhorn, August. *Wayward Youth*. New York: Viking Press, 1974/1925.

American Psychiatric Association. *A Psychiatric Glossary: The Meaning of Terms Frequently Used in Psychiatry, 4th Edition*. Washington, DC: American Psychiatric Association Publications Office, 1975.

American Psychiatric Association. *Diagnostic and Statistical Manual of Mental Disorders, 5th Edition*. Washington, DC: American Psychiatric Association, 2013.

Bakhtin, Mikhail. *Rabelais and His World*. Translated by Helene Iswolsky. Bloomington, IN: Indiana University Press, 1984.

Barthes, Roland. "The Metaphor of the Eye." In *Critical Essays*, 239–248. Edited and translated by Richard Howard. Evanston, IL: Northwestern University Press, 1992.

Bataille, Georges. "Un-knowing: Laughter and Tears." In *October*, 89–102. Vol. 36, 1986a/1953.

Bataille, Georges. *Erotism: Death & Sensuality*. Translated by Mary Dalwood. San Francisco, CA: City Lights Books, 1986b/1957.

Bataille, Georges. *The Story of the Eye*. Translated by Joachim Neugroschel. San Francisco, CA: City Lights Books, 1987/1928.

Bataille, Georges. "Solar Anus." In *Visions of Excess: Selected Writings, 1927–1939*, 5–9. Edited and translated by Allan Stoekl. Minneapolis, MN: University of Minnesota Press, 1991a/1927.

Bataille, Georges. "Eye." In *Visions of Excess: Selected Writings, 1927–1939*, 17–19. Edited and translated by Allan Stoekl. Minneapolis, MN: University of Minnesota Press, 1991b/1929.

Bataille, Georges. "Rotten sun." In *Visions of Excess: Selected Writings, 1927–1939*, 57–58. Edited and translated by Allan Stoekl. Minneapolis, MN: University of Minnesota Press, 1991c/1930.

Bataille, Georges. "Mouth." In *Visions of Excess: Selected Writings, 1927–1939*, 59–60. Edited and translated by Allan Stoekl. Minneapolis, MN: University of Minnesota Press, 1991d/1930.

Bataille, Georges. "Sacrificial Mutilation and the Severed Ear of Vincent Van Gogh." In *Visions of Excess: Selected Writings, 1927–1939*, 61–72. Edited and translated by Allan Stoekl. Minneapolis, MN: University of Minnesota Press, 1991e/1930.

Bataille, Georges. "The Jesuve." In *Visions of Excess: Selected Writings, 1927–1939*, 73–78. Edited and translated by Allan Stoekl. Minneapolis, MN: University of Minnesota Press, 1991f/1930.

Bataille, Georges. "The Use Value of D. A. F. de Sade (An Open Letter to My Current Comrades)." In *Visions of Excess: Selected Writings, 1927–1939*, 91–102. Edited and translated by Allan Stoekl. Minneapolis, MN: University of Minnesota Press, 1991g/1930.

Bataille, Georges. "The Notion of Expenditure." In *Visions of Excess: Selected Writings, 1927–1939*, 116–129. Edited and translated by Allan Stoekl. Minneapolis, MN: University of Minnesota Press, 1991h/1933.

Bataille, Georges. "The Pineal Eye." In *Visions of Excess: Selected Writings, 1927–1939*, 79–90. Edited and translated by Allan Stoekl. Minneapolis, MN: University of Minnesota Press, 1991i/1967.

Bataille, Georges. *The Accursed Share: An Essay on General Economy, Volume 1*. Translated by Robert Hurley. New York: Zone Books, 1991j/1967.

Bataille, Georges. *The Accursed Share: An Essay on General Economy, Volumes II and III*. Translated by Robert Hurley. New York: Zone Books, 1991k/1976.

Benjamin, Walter. "The Work of Art in the Age of Its Technological Reproducibility." In *Walter Benjamin: Selected Writings, Vol. 4, 1938–1940*, 251–283. Translated by Edmund Jephcott; Edited by Howard Eiland and Michael W. Jennings. Cambridge, MA: Belknap Press, 2003/1939.

Blondel, Eric. *Nietzsche, The Body and Culture: Philosophy as a Philological Genealogy*. Translated by Sean Hand. Stanford, CA: Stanford University Press, 1991.

Blos, Peter. *On Adolescence: A Psychoanalytic Interpretation*. New York: Free Press, 1967.

Breton, Andre. *Mad Love*. Translated by Mary Ann Caws. Lincoln, NE: University of Nebraska Press, Bison Books, 1988/1937.

Canetti, Elias. *Crowds and Power*. Translated by Carol Stewart. New York: Noonday Press, 1993.

Cullen, Deborah (ed.). "Interview: Deborah Cullen by Noam Chasin." In *Bataille's Eye: Institute of Cultural Inquiry, Field Notes*, 10–19. Vol. 4, 1997.

Douglas, Mary. *Purity and Danger: An Analysis of Concepts of Pollution and Taboo*. New York: Penguin Books, 1970.

Evans, Douglas. "Metonymy." In *An Introductory Dictionary of Lacanian Psychoanalysis*, 113–114. Edited by Deborah Cullen. New York: Routledge, 1996.

Fenichel, Otto. "The Scoptophilic Instinct and Identification." In *The Collected Papers of Otto Fenichel, First Series*, 373–397. Collected and edited by Hanna Fenichel and David Rapaport. New York: W. W. Norton & Company, 1953.

Fenichel, Otto. "Neurotic Acting Out." In *The Collected Papers of Otto Fenichel, Second Series*, 296–304. Collected and edited by Hanna Fenichel and David Rapaport. New York: W. W. Norton & Company, 1954.

Ferenczi, Sandor. "Laughter." In *Final Contributions to the Problems and Methods of Psychoanalysis*, 177–182. Edited by Ernest Jones. New York: Brunner/Mazel, 1980a/1913.

Ferenczi, Sandor. "The Ontogenesis of the Interest in Money." In *First Contributions to Psychoanalysis*. Edited and translated by Ernest Jones. New York: Brunner/Mazel Publishers, 1980b/1914.

Fleiss, Robert. *Erogeneity and Libido: Some Addenda to the Theory of the Psychosexual Development of the Human*. New York: International Universities Press, 1956.

Foster, Hal. *Convulsive Beauty*. Cambridge, MA: MIT Press, 1993.

Freud, Sigmund. "Three Essays on the Theory of Sexuality." In *The Standard Edition of the Complete Psychological Works of Sigmund Freud, Volume VII*, 125–248. Edited and translated by James Strachey. London: Hogarth Press, 1957a/1905.

Freud, Sigmund. "Three Psychoanalytic View of Psychogenic Disturbance of Vision." In *The Standard Edition of the Complete Psychological Works of Sigmund Freud, Volume XI*, 209–218. Edited and translated by James Strachey. London: Hogarth Press, 1957b/1910.

Freud, Sigmund. "Character and Anal Erotism." In *The Standard Edition of the Complete Psychological Works of Sigmund Freud, Volume IX*, 167–176. Edited and translated by James Strachey. London: Hogarth Press, 1959/1908.

Freud, Sigmund. "Civilization and its Discontents." In *The Standard Edition of the Complete Psychological Works of Sigmund Freud, Volume XXI*, 59–148. Edited and translated by James Strachey. London: Hogarth Press, 1961/1930.

Greenson, Ralph, R. *The Technique and Practice of Psychoanalysis, Volume 1*. New York: International Universities Press, 1979.

Griaule, Marcel. "Eye (3. Evil Eye)." In *Encyclopedia Acephalica*, 47–48. Edited by Georges Bataille. Translated by Iain White. London: Atlas Press, 1995/1929.

Guntrip, Harry. *Personality Structure and Human Interaction: The Developing Synthesis of Psycho-dynamic Theory*. New York: International Universities Press, 1961.

Heimann, Paula. "Notes on the Anal Stage." In *About Children and Children-No-Longer, Collected Papers 1942–80*, 169–184. Edited by Margret Tonnesmann. New York: Tavistock/Routledge, 1989/1961.

Jacobson, Edith. *The Self and the Object World*. New York: International Universities Press, 1964.

Jay, Martin. *Downcast Eyes: The Denigration of Vision in Twentieth-century French Thought*. Berkeley, CA: University of California Press, 1994.

Kendall, Stuart. "Making More (of Waste)." In *Georges Bataille and Contemporary Thought*, 73–94. Edited by Will Stronge. New York: Bloomsbury Academic, 2019.

Klein, Melanie. *Love, Guilt, and Reparation & Other Works, 1921–1945*. New York: Delta Books, 1977/1936.

Kohut, Heinz. *The Analysis of the Self: A Systematic Approach to the Treatment of Narcissistic Personality Disorders*. New York: International Universities Press, 1969.

Krauss, Rosalind. "Photography in the Service of Surrealism." In *L'Amour Fou*, 15–56. Edited by Rosalind Krauss and Jane Livingston. New York: Abbeville Press, 1985.

Krauss, Rosalind E. *The Optical Unconscious*. Cambridge, MA: MIT Press, 1993.

Kristeva, Julia. *Powers of Horror: An Essay on Abjection*. Translated by Leon S. Roudiez. New York: Columbia University Press, 1982.

Kussel, Peter B. "From the Anus to the Mouth to the Eye." In *Semiotext(e)*, 105–120. Vol. II (2), 1976.

Lacan, Jacques. "From Anal to Ideal." In *Anxiety: The Seminar of Jacques Lacan, Book X*, 294–309. Edited by Jacques-Alain Miller. Translated by A. R. Price. Malden, MA: Polity Press, 2018/1963.

Langs, Robert. *The Therapeutic Interaction: A Synthesis*. New York: Jason Aronson, Inc., 1977.

LaPlanche, Jean and Pontalis, J.-B. *The Language of Psychoanalysis*. Translated by Donald Nicholson-Smith. New York: W. W. Norton & Company, 1973.

Malinowski, Bronisław. *Argonauts of the Western Pacific: An Account of the Native Enterprise and Adventure in the Archipelagoes of Melanesia New Guinea*. New York: E. P. Dutton & Company, 1961.

Mauss, Marcel. *The Gift: Forms and Functions of Exchange in Archaic Societies*. Translated by Ian Cunnison. New York: W. W. Norton & Company, 1967/1925.

McWilliams, Nancy. *Psychoanalytic Diagnosis: Understanding Personality Structure in the Clinical Process*. New York: Guilford Press, 1994.

Meissner, W. W. *Internalization in Psychoanalysis*. New York: International Universities Press, 1981.

Miller, William I. *The Anatomy of Disgust*. Cambridge, MA: Harvard University Press, 1997.

Ogden, Thomas. "On Projective Identification." In *International Journal of Psychoanalysis*, 357–373. Vol. 60, 1979.

Partridge, Eric. *Origins: A Short Etymological Dictionary of Modern English, 2nd Edition*. New York: Macmillan Company, 1959.

Reich, Annie. *Psychoanalytic Contributions*. New York: International Universities Press, 1973.

Rose, Jacqueline. *Sexuality in the Field of Vision*. New York: Verso. 1996.

Schilder, Paul. *The Image and Appearance of the Human Body: Studies in the Constructive Energies of the Psyche*. New York: International Universities Press, 1978.

Segal, Hanna. *Introduction to the Work of Melanie Klein, 2nd Edition*. New York: Basic Books, 1974.

Stallybrass, Peter & Allon White. *The Politics and Poetics of Transgression*. Ithaca, NY: Cornell University Press, 1992.

Stoekl, Allan. *Bataille's Peak: Energy, Religion, and Postsustainability*. Minneapolis, MN: University of Minnesota Press, 2007.

Strachey, James. "The Nature of the Therapeutic Action of Psycho-analysis." In *International Journal of Psychoanalysis*, 127–159. Vol. 15, 1934.

Winnicott, Donald. "Fear of Breakdown." In *International Revue of Psychoanalysis*, 103–107. Vol. 1, 1974.

Winnicott, Donald. "The Antisocial Tendency." In *Through Pediatrics to Psychoanalysis*, 306–315. New York: Basic Books, 1975.

Winnicott, Donald. "The Use of an Object and Relating Through Identifications." In *Playing and Reality*, 101–111. Edited by M. Masud R. Khan. New York: Penguin Books, 1980.

Winnicott, Donald. "The Theory of the Parent-infant Relationship." In *The Maturational Processes and the Facilitating Environment: Studies in the Theory of Emotional Development*. Edited by M. Masud R. Khan. Madison, CT: International Universities Press, 1991/1960.

Chapter 6

The accursed child

With Pony[1]

The theater of cruelty wants a dance
of eyelids coupled up with elbows and kneecaps
and femurs and toes,
and wills it seen.

Antonin Artaud (1947)

Pony was the only child born to a couple whose ability to love and care for each other, much less her, proved to be fleeting, transitory, and unsustainable. In lieu of adequate parental caretaking, her need for a sense of belonging and affiliation was left, by default, to the motley group of extended relatives with whom she shared a home. It was in this early state of emotional neglect that her uncle C found her, perhaps owing to his own sense of marginalization within the family. The common element of being lost and neglected within the family home was the basis from which they each felt found together. And the power of being found in this way was paradisiacal. Never before or since had the experience of being seen and loved meant so much ... (Pony: *My friend, you show your hand in this ellipsis. When you described your transit through the bog-like field of my internal world as moonless dark, I understood it to be a kind of willful blindness. For sure as I have lit my own way with the frightful lightning of nightmare and the burning of my own body, I have shown my hand to you time after time. We reject that which is closest, for those things are near enough to burn. To say 'never since' is a disservice to the work we do, don't you think? If transference is the final stage of our work together, then*

---

1 Prefatory note: this document is an artifact of an active treatment process. As such, it is intended primarily for the therapeutic benefit of Pony, the subject of this treatment, and secondarily for the reader who is seeking to understand the process from a distance. It consists of five sources of information: the author/therapist's narrative; Pony's parenthetical, italicized commentary on the narrative; emails from Pony; drawings from Pony; and photographs by/from Pony and the author. It charts a journey, by way of dialogical collaboration, whose arrival in form is itself the intended therapeutic goal.

aren't you called now to own the love he so greedily drank up before the shame of it destroyed the both of us? For what is love if not the closest we can come to being known?)

And then, as quickly as it emerged, it was over. In the first of a series of events that dissolved any fledgling sense of belonging, her parents moved her away from the close proximity to family; friends; and, especially, her uncle. This move was followed by the separation of her parents, who divorced shortly after, and the mysterious illness and death of her uncle at a young age. Inexplicably evicted from any familiar sense of home, family, and self, her radical estrangement left her again existentially experiencing herself and the world as formless. (Pony: *'Formless,' though I accept the term in this context, implies something indistinct. In fact, what I experienced was terrifyingly distinct, if obscured, if symbolic. My experience of self is only formless in the sense that it endlessly transfigures out of necessity ... No, the things that plagued me were distinct. The specter of violence was so clear to me that I feared it could take me or those around me at any moment. And it took. It took my grandfather, which took the last of my mother's kindness. It took my pets and the animals that lived in my neighborhood. I gathered their bodies when I could and buried them under a tree in the yard, dead birds and squirrels and my rabbits and sometimes even plants, flower heads knocked off the stems, because I couldn't bear to look at them, because I was so jealous of their freedom and of the power that took them, a power that I was too afraid to wield.*) Yet now her pain was compounded by having known love and lost it so dramatically. Why had this happened? In that imaginative direction toward which isolated children are so easily inclined, she wondered what she had done wrong. What transgression resulted in the fall of her family and the loss of the only love she could trust? (Pony: *In the end, I had always known that it was my responsibility. To complete the interrupted work that had begun when I myself was in the process of forming.*)

Consciously, Pony sought help managing a debilitating depression from which there seemed no relief – becoming older and moving out into the world only meant increasing consciousness of being Other, the experience that had plagued her for so long that it felt intrinsically synonymous with Self. However, unconsciously, Pony came to me seeking expiation for a sin she could not remember. A sin that, once remembered and named, would explain her marginalization and the chronic mental and physical unease that accompanied it. (Pony: *Is 'unease' adequate to describe the agony that remains a constant feature of my life?*)

From the outset psychotherapeutic treatment had the reconnaissance task of finding Pony. This was not simply a matter of entering the collapsed mine of the depressive experience, so to speak, in order to dig out with the patient (metaphorical analogy from Levenson 1972). (Pony: *This line recalled one of my most frightening recurring nightmares: Down a dirt road, a rotting shack with an opening in the ground. Down the opening, a long and dirty corridor where chicken wire cages contained stacks and rows of malformed, tortured animals. I struggled to free them, though their appearance was so disturbing that I could scarcely look at them. All the while, the fear that the farmer, sometimes imagined as a scientist, [for I never looked at him directly] would catch me trying to free them and I would die; though I also knew that I would die if I didn't free them.*) Rather it would require entering a landscape who's only defining characteristic is formlessness (I refer here to Bataille's (1991a, 31) notion of formlessness in which signification, and "what it designates has no rights in any sense and gets itself squashed everywhere, like a spider or an earthworm"). How would one empathically enter this experience as anything but a bull in a china shop, insisting, however subtly, that verbally naming her experience will be therapeutic because it "serves to bring things down in the world, generally requiring that each thing have its form" (31)? Surely this would require more than Freud's technical recommendation to psychoanalysts for a stance of "evenly suspended attention" (Freud 1958c, 111). Rather, I adopted Bion's (1981) technical recommendation as more fitted to my task:

> Every session attended by the psychoanalyst must have no history and no future. What is 'known' about the patient is of no further consequence: it is either false or irrelevant. If it is 'known' by patient and analyst, it is obsolete … The only point of importance in any session is the unknown. Nothing must be allowed to distract from that. In any session, evolution takes place. Out of the darkness and formlessness something evolves. That evolution can bear a superficial resemblance to memory, but once it has been experienced it can never be confounded with memory. It shares with dreams the quality of being wholly present or unaccountably and suddenly absent. The evolution is what the psychoanalyst must be ready to interpret.
> 260

Experiencing formlessness together in therapy became the project which, perhaps predictably, inevitably, was destined to transferentially retrace the earlier path taken by Pony and her uncle. (Which is to say, I expected that, "the impulses and feelings directed toward the analyst were, thus, *transferred* from the original objects" Racker 1991, 13, author's emphasis).

From the first session Pony presented as an exceptionally attractive and intelligent, petite woman who appeared much younger than her 23 years. She was already an accomplished musician after years of conservatory training. However, her creative resources extended well beyond music as she had also been drawing, painting, and writing since early childhood. Her extraordinary talent would be a greater source of pleasure but for the fact that she did not trust people enough to internalize their consistent praise of her. Performance, in every aspect of her life, seemed to strangely serve both expressive and defensive purposes.

Our starting point, as per the usual custom in any treatment, was Pony's conscious presenting problem: her lifelong creative expression was blocked. She knew something was seriously wrong when her familiar self-sustaining activities of drawing and writing simply stopped. She was numb to the point of being expressionless, even for herself. Whatever part of Pony that was available to observe her own predicament realized then that this unprecedented paralysis of her usually florid visual and literary expression, this "phantasmatic inhibition," spelt trouble (Kristeva 1995, 10). This is what prompted her contacting me to commence treatment. It directly and indirectly determined the focus, the trajectory, and the goal of our work, that is, to recover her zest, her verve for the praxis of self-representation.

I came to learn that Pony moved through her days with an especially disturbing, visceral experience of dread. (Pony: *To illustrate, the dread was not without form. To drive in traffic is to imagine mangled cars and bodies smeared across the pavement. To visit a cousin with a new baby, to have the baby placed in my arms is to experience with painful clarity the waking dream with all the sense data of real life [sound and smell and weight and texture and vivid sight] in which I drop the baby and its brains splash across the floor.)* So severe was this that her chronic psychological experience of unease seemed to manifest as disease; she developed, at a relatively young age, symptoms related to Rheumatoid Arthritis along with chronic stomach pain. This was further compounded by bouts of anxiety, depression, emotional darkness, and dissociation. The combination of physical symptoms and lost history cumulatively contributed to the unrelenting experience of being disoriented and out-of-place in her body and in the world. Her amnesia for the early experience that both protected her and precluded relief, plagued her every day. So we together agreed to set about trying to put together the clues that might reveal the knowledge that would finally release her.

Gradually, slowly, Pony moved into the dark past. There was the girl that lived nearby in the neighborhood who asked her to play only to direct her on how to masturbate with a stuffed animal; meanwhile the ominous shadow of the girl's older brother loomed in the background but remained undefined. There was also the striking (on recollection) fascination with graphic pornography. (Pony: *Again, to clarify, that the things which drew me were not only explicit but necessarily violent, to the point of simulated torture and death.)* And then there was the week when she adamantly insisted that her mother refer to her only as Dorothy (from the Wizard of Oz); (Pony: *For a long time I had considered it a betrayal that Dorothy was sent back over the rainbow at the end.)* the desperate insistence of this command led her mother to bring Pony to a psychotherapist at an early age for an abbreviated treatment that included drawing and coloring (see Figure 6.1). These and other recollections functioned for us as smoke signaling fire. However, two additional features of her childhood stood out most prominently, in part because both had endured into the present. These were her social marginalization and her affinity for animals.

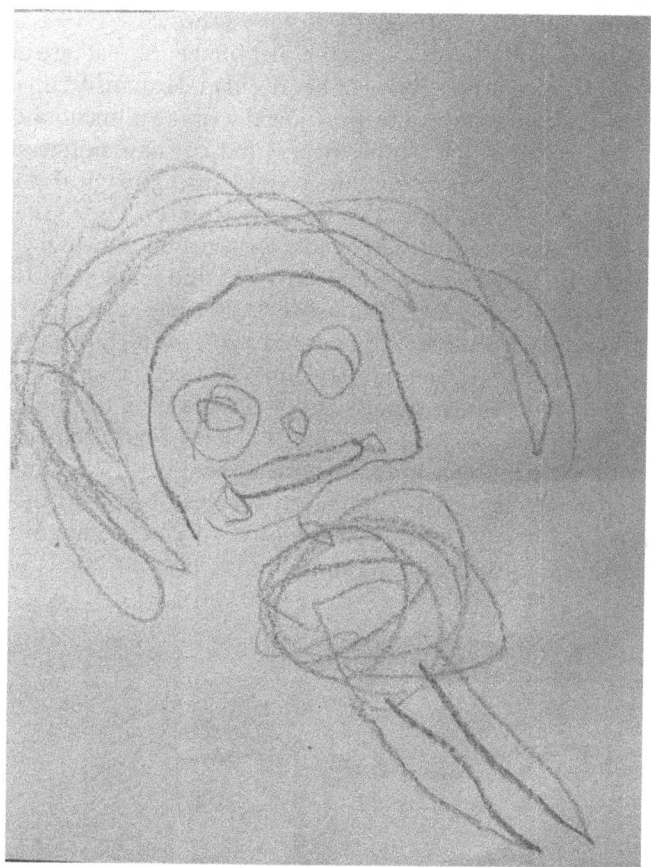

Figure 6.1 An early childhood drawing while "in treatment."
Source: All photographs taken by the author except where otherwise indicated.

Throughout childhood Pony felt utterly different from other children. It was as though she participated in another culture whose emotional language she did not understand. This motivated Pony to a level of academic performance that was extraordinary; where her best efforts failed with her peers, she might at least ingratiate herself to her teachers. She could best approach something resembling social validation only with adults – a further sign arousing her suspicion in recollection. The pain of being socially ostracized was intolerable and led to her choking a classmate that she felt was looking at her disapprovingly. (Pony: *Though this memory is a bad one for the shame that followed, the moment in which I put my hands around her throat was transcendent; it was a rare moment of relief at a time when my distress was heightened. This was shortly after Uncle C died.*) This particular event landed her in the principal's office thus exacerbating her sense of marginalization and undermining her efforts at even the adult's approval.

The consequence of Pony's loneliness was her further retreat into an interior world within the safe, relative control of her florid and expansive imagination. That world was not characterized by the typical wish-fulfillment tales of most people (see Freud 1959). In fact, other people did not have admittance there at all. Rather, it was a mythopoetic universe featuring magical powers and animals as spirit guardians. From this fertile place grew Pony's lifelong love of animals as well as the fine arts, especially writing and drawing.

Perhaps more than anything, animals invoked and made manifest Pony's magical world. Not for the sake of inventing alternate, different, or better categories of human life. Rather, Pony might agree with Haraway (2008, 19) who declared "I am not a posthumanist; I am who I become with companion species, who and which makes a mess out of categories in the making of kin and kind. Queer messmates in mortal play, indeed." Thus, Pony had always shared her life with rabbits, horses, guinea pigs, cats, dogs, fish, birds, etc. Nor was her menagerie of companion species limited to these actual domestic animals. Through her zoomorphic artwork her companion species included the therianthropic, or human-animal hybrids (see Figure 6.2).

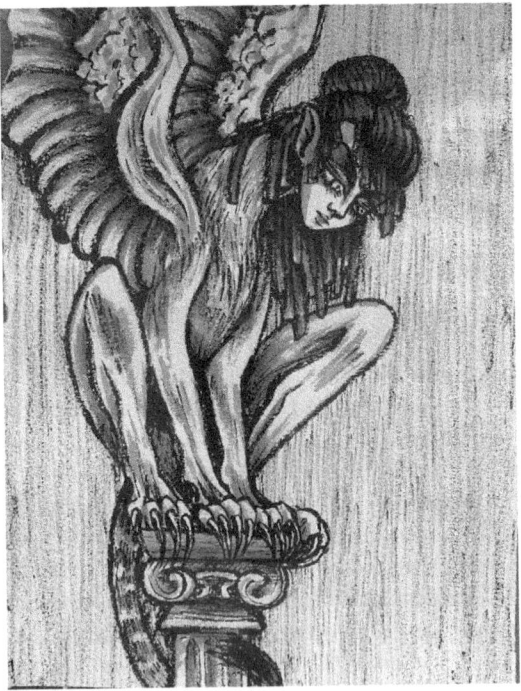

Figure 6.2 Therianthropic self-representation.

Many of her drawings were self-representations that demonstrated a nascent shamanic sensibility (I will return to the subject of shamanic identity later).

With animals, real and imagined, Pony was not painfully Other but at ease in communion. This could be construed as anti-social or anti-humanist but it was more particular than that. The medium of communication with animals was always non-verbal, sometimes physical, and always intuitive. (Pony: *I will say that while I vividly remember Uncle C's voice, I only remember it as he spoke to others. Ours was a secret language of glance and touch. I felt and still feel that to speak is to translate. The deep joy of my time riding horses was that of speaking in one's native tongue at last after a long time in exile.*) Without language and all the categorical, conceptual thinking it implies – past/future, good/bad, inner/outer – Pony could safely resort to "the radical possibilities of communication through silence" (Richman 2017, 157). In other words, it was that communication that, predicated on silence, exists pre-form, in formlessness. In adulthood Pony would experience a variant of this type of connection in her strikingly successful work tutoring autistic children, a population she had a special affinity for given her facility for non-verbal, intuitive communication.

With independent living looming following her graduation, Pony was confronted with yet another loss of community and structure that sent her into an even deeper, darker emotional state. All options involving dependence on others – whether family, friends, or teachers – seemed impossible. Her physical symptoms related to RA worsened and the medication only seemed to compound it. She grew increasingly despondent. For several cold, winter months she house-sat in a distant New York suburb alone with only a friend's dog to keep her company. Our weekly phone sessions seemed insufficiently sustaining; Pony was confronted with the task of speaking to an experience that either resisted words or that existed before words. We could not be sure. Yet it seemed increasingly likely that the darkness, fear, and dread descending on her was correlated with our continuous efforts to uncover/ recover the memories that she believed would explain her pain.

In this darkest hour Pony, as much from desperation as from calculation, and trusting an uncanny intuition that had always been her one and only reliable guide, embarked on a series of bold moves. She decided to end her isolation despite her anxiety about others and move back into the city where she could live and interact with people. Pony also decided to turn her back on a certain career in music in favor of a career as a tattoo artist. (Pony: *For as long as I can remember, there was a certain horror around being seen. The silent observer followed me always through my day, as I dressed, as I ate, as I tried to play. It could see through walls and under all my clothes and it watched me when I bathed, when I used the toilet. There was refuge in water – particularly the sea, and I spent a lot of time in and around the ocean as a child. Uncle C would often take me to the duck pond to feed stale Wonder bread to the ducks and geese, and I envied their easy transit to the unreachable water, out into the pond where people couldn't cross. Of course, they could; the pond was just a pond. But the easy slip from land to water, to a secretive place [it seems to me that birds are so secretive in their unreachable nests] was enviable. Who would want to fly in open sky? I wanted the water, the glasslike barrier with its hidden murk. I dreamed of them often, featherless and embryonic, suspended in the endless dark. A stage is a liminal place. But looking inward made a burden of illusion. I think that if I had never looked too far inside, if I never broke the surface of memory for what hid beneath, I could have been a powerful performer. So many unnamed pains funneled out through that illusion – 'perché me ne rimuneri così?' But by naming, by looking in, the spell was broken, the barrier gone. And all I could see anymore was a hundred eyes watching, not the illusion, but me. I couldn't bear it.)*

Her talent, beauty, and intelligence attracted all types of attention walking into her first tattoo parlor job. She was quickly recruited by a more experienced male tattoo artist, E, who served, as is the professional custom, as her mentor. An intimacy ensued that she had not known in a very long time. In this regard it is worth noting that her new mentor E reminded her, in his physical appearance at least, of her late uncle. (Pony: *What sold me on E was the hands. He had large hands, rough from the punishment of climbing chain link and concrete. He was a graffiti writer, so his hands were always flecked with paint. Uncle C did a lot of odd jobs when I was a child but worked primarily as a house painter. His hands were always rough and always flecked with paint.*) Under his tutelage Pony quickly and easily developed her confidence and reputation in the shop. However, perhaps even more important were the nocturnal trips they made to train yards in and around the city to paint, graffiti-style, on the sides of trains and other public surfaces – in the dark, in silence, and in fear of being caught. (Pony: *I cannot begin to express the impression my time as a writer left on me. It's the nearest thing to magic I've ever experienced in sober, waking life. To be born as a writer is to be born new, over and over and over again. I, alone, creating myself from nothing, saying I am I am I am, pony pony pony pony pony.*) Her graffiti art would eventually earn her the name "Pony" in the graffiti community, and this name became the personal signature of her work (see Figure 6.3).

The combination of finding special attention and secretive shared danger with a man that closely resembled her uncle was pulling us closer, however unconsciously, to the truth she withheld from herself.

During this period, and still in a strong surge of self-determination, Pony attended an ayahuasca session with the hope of revelation and healing. (Despite the critique of casual, nonnativist ayahuasca use (see Taussig and Wilson 2002), ayahuasca is being increasingly regarded as a healing option for trauma in contemporary urban society beyond the legitimation of either anthropology or modern medicine (Ott 1996; Walsh and Grob 2005). This intuitive, last ditch conscious effort at an answer to her mystery was rewarded. Her first experience was highly peculiar in that she experienced

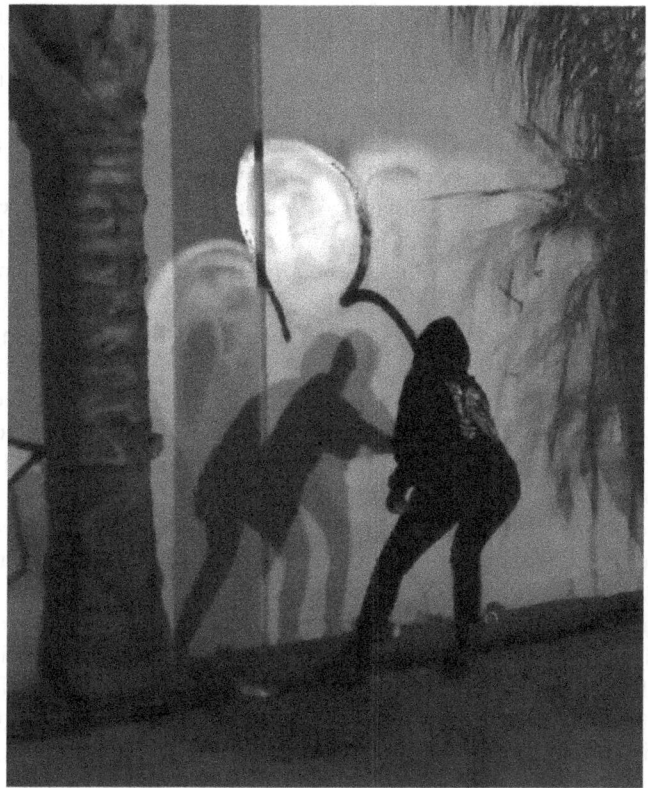

Figure 6.3 Pony drawing "like Peter Pan and his shadow."

none of the usual purging associated with the entheogen. Instead, Pony experienced with conviction the horrifying answer she had been denying herself for years – it was her uncle who had engaged her in far-reaching sexual interaction from the time she was four years old.

How had ayahuasca succeeded where years of therapy had failed to uncover the traumatic past? I contend that nothing short of an altered state of consciousness was required in order to access the repressed memory. (Pony: *It is my sincere [naive] hope that none of you are ever forced to understand the difficulty with which I handle these experiences with their sense-memory pressed in chaotic and harrowing detail into the very fiber of my body. You could not possibly know without experiencing such a thing firsthand. No pain I've experienced since has ever come close.*) Not only for the reasons Freud and Breuer (1957) describe in their clinical work with hypnosis, but because the trance state best approximates the state of Pony during which she first experienced the traumatic sexual acts as a child. What is crucial is *"the level of consciousness at which the content is apprehended"* (Wolinsky 1991, 25, author's emphasis). Of course, like the recovered early memories of Freud's and Breuer's patients, Pony's recollection in an altered state is open to critical dispute as to whether it is a product of historical or narrative truth (on the importance of this distinction see Spence 1982; Masson 1984; Crews 1995). That is, disputed in the same way as are the accounts of illness diagnosed and healed by shamans in an altered state through feats of transubstantiation, transfiguration, and possession. However, the therapeutic value, if not the veracity of a clinical narrative, should not be assessed from a perspective outside the altered state of consciousness from which it was experienced. Moreover, ayahuasca was particularly suited to Pony's exploration of trauma to the extent that it "brings out and indeed depends upon intense living at extremity and exploration of the inchoate" (Taussig 1991, 406). If I were in need of corroborating evidence for the original events as recalled by Pony, I witnessed her abreaction in front of me as confirmation: Pony's RA symptoms left almost immediately as did her interpersonal symptoms related to depression.

Her revelation hit like an explosive and accordingly illuminated several dark corners of her attenuated childhood and adolescence. Suddenly, all at once, the years of feeling Other with family and peers which culminated in a deep distrust of human intimacy all made sense. The early mysterious death of her uncle following his withdrawal from Pony now seemed more like a guilt-ridden self-imposed exile after he realized his atrocious exploitation. Pony struggled to digest the new information. Several sessions were dominated by her plaintive and wailing plea that I explain how a grown man could even consider such an act. Now more than ever the slightest suggestion of any and all sexuality from men she encountered was threatening and highly suspect. The adamant determination to reclaim her own body was paramount and received major impetus from her growing involvement with body art. And yet this reaction to the memory of her uncle and his appropriation of her unwitting sexual participation as a child was only one aspect of what developed.

Pony also came to understand her furious contempt and disgust for her childhood caretakers. How were they so ignorant? How did they not see what was happening right in front of them? (Pony: *I am at risk of appearing hysterical when I say that it's happened in front of you too. In the same way you turn your eyes from the unsightly figure of the homeless and forget them not minutes later, you turn your eyes from me, even as I play with your children, with your nieces and nephews. Even as I cry to you with what limited language I have, you, who should know, turn away and forget not minutes later. You remember me in a guilty flash days or weeks later just to push the image away with a shrug. What can you do? What can you do? You cannot know what it means to a person in need just to simply be seen. See me in that moment. See my pain, it's the least you can do.*) Confronting her parents today with the facts of her abuse back then initially met with denial or worse, indifference.

This served only to confirm her early experience of neglect that left her susceptible to her uncle in the first place. These and more questions led only to illogical answers and a horror, rage, and deep distrust of a society where a child could be so terribly exploited in plain sight. It was only when considering the work of Georges Bataille that I glimpsed, at least hypothetically, the perverse explanation for the behavior of her family.

Pony's family was overtly identified with their Italian ancestral legacy. This included a strong, if nondevout, awareness of their Roman Catholic heritage. From this perspective, at least in the Italian-American cultural context of the late twentieth century in Northern New Jersey, female sexuality was a nonerotic event for procreation incumbent on the married couple of the household in order to expand the clan. "Frequently, young Italian women say that their adult status was not really accepted by their parents, even after career and marital success, until they produced children themselves" (Giordano and McGoldrick 1996, 573). The Roman Catholic view of women alternated between saints and whores with a virgin birth depicted as the pinnacle of piety. Moreover, the ultimate act of ecstatic salvation was a human sacrifice. I imagined the horror of being, as Bataille would put it, the accursed female child sacrificed by the family for the appeasement of a frightening male God of retribution. Would the gift of this little girl make her uncle whole again? Would it finally transform him into the kind of man who could fulfill his cultural obligation? (Pony: *Uncle C neither dated, even as a young man, nor married, and lived with my grandparents till the day he died. He appeared to the family obstinately opposed to romance. How little they knew. He was one of eight children and [barring S who died before he was old enough to be bothered about it] all the others married and had children. Couldn't keep track of all of them, my grandmother used to joke. He fell through, another domino, him and then me.*) Further into the treatment Pony revealed to me numerous other incestuously abusive situations involving her mother and grandfather as well as within the families of several of her cousins.

Two more ayahuasca sessions went a long way toward empowering Pony. Her encounter with the spirit animals and plants of these adventures were especially helpful due to her pre-existing rapport with and proclivity for non-human forms of life. She was aided in her ayahuasca quest by the guidance of a cougar and a white snake. These highly affirming and healing experiences notwithstanding, we repeatedly came back to her uncle. He was executed and disposed of again and again during her ayahuasca sessions as well as in fantasy, and yet he did not leave. We gradually came to the most painful recollection of all. Painful, that is, in that it consisted of very complicated positive and special feelings she held for her uncle that she could not/did not want to extinguish.

Pony and her uncle were very close prior to the introduction of sex into their relationship. He had seen her as special in ways that her own parents missed. His birthday and Christmas gifts reflected the love of a man who actually listened to her and cared how she felt. In her eyes, he was admirable and charismatic. Moreover, with time, Pony came to see her uncle and herself as similar. Her love and need for his love flourished through a "confusion of tongues" into a full identification with him (see Ferenczi 1980, for a clear exposition on how this type of identification develops).

Finally, after weeks of our highly tentative discussion of this positive side of the relationship she was able to admit an even deeper truth. Perhaps it was not the sex between them that was most traumatic, it was that he dropped her and walked out of her life as she grew older and matured into a highly articulate intelligent girl. (Pony: *If I never hear the word 'precocious' ever again, I would be glad. I potty trained young because I hated to be touched, to have my legs lifted up, to be looked at like that. I learned to speak young and I learned to read young, and I learned words from TV and the world around me and they all seemed afraid, because suddenly I could name the parts that I didn't want them to touch anymore.*) As excruciatingly painful as intercourse with an adult was at such a tender age, it was being abandoned in the aftermath, after giving everything of herself, that she could not fathom or recover from. This abrupt abandonment was central to the etiology of her self-loathing. At a crucial formative period of her life, the same person who had made her feel special, albeit at a traumatic cost, also left her feeling worthless. Moreover, her revelation and discussion of their sexual relationship with me constituted a betrayal of their pact; according to her uncle she was never to tell anyone of their physical relationship for fear of her parents' dying. Thus, a debilitating equation was established early on between open sharing and destruction and this had ramifications for our therapy.

> Italian families are full of 'secrets,' as the therapist will soon learn by asking a question that is out of bounds. The existence of secrets may be puzzling to the therapist since the family seems to talk openly about all kinds of issues, including sex, bodily functions, and hostility … Therapists must deal delicately with secrets, being aware of the sense of betrayal families will feel if the line is crossed.
>
> Giordano and McGoldrick (1996, 577)

Beyond the ominous threat against disclosing her secret, there exists the cultural equation of a secret with sin; disclosure or abreaction with confession; and even, perversely, abreaction with sin: "abreaction is also the discharge between language and act" (Cixous and Clement 1986, 16).

To express feelings regarding her uncle that were particularly painful and complicated Pony resorted to email "letters" like the following (edited) messages that she sent me between sessions:

> It's crazy to me how similar we are. I look like him. We make the same facial expressions. There's one look in particular I'm wearing in a majority

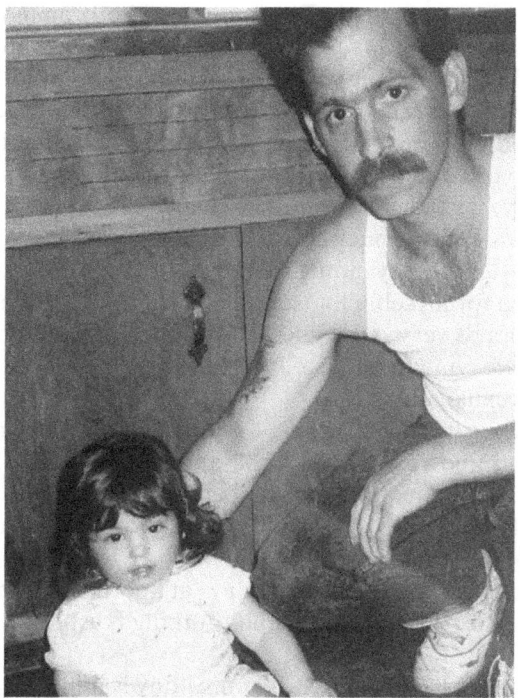

Figure 6.4 "The face of knowing too much."

of the photos of me as a child. I think it's the face of knowing too much. Or maybe it's the face of being overwhelmed. He wears the same face in the picture of us where he's wearing the purple jeans [see Figure 6.4].

There are very few pictures of me and my father, and almost all of them are from holidays. There are basically no pictures of me and my mother.

After we moved away from him there's a big gap where there's hardly any pictures of me at all – only school pictures, or staged ones like the one with the bunny.

That's around the time I had a dissociative episode that lasted upwards of two weeks, where I wouldn't respond to my own name but insisted I was Dorothy from the Wizard of Oz. Some child psychologist that cleared me after that one.

You can see in the bunny picture there's a little ring around my lower lip. A red crescent shape right underneath my lip. I was having nightmares very badly during this time, and I was very anxious during the day. I would bite my lower lip until it bled, all day long, even though it hurt. I couldn't help myself. I had that crescent mark for most of the school year.

Thumper died in my arms. We didn't have him very long. My parents didn't clean his cage enough. The poop would pile up in the corner – he was smart and only pooped in one corner. But it piled up too much and his little tail was constantly caked in it, so he got an infection. He got sick, and I woke up one day to find him seizing up in the corner of the cage. I picked him up and my dad drove us to the vet but he died in my arms as we parked in the vet's office. That was a tough one.

I was six years old. My grandfather died later that year, my uncle's father. It was all pretty much constant chaos after that – not that it wasn't before. But after that my mom fell apart for real. My dad checked out for real. I cooked for myself a lot (scrambled eggs made in the microwave).

This all sounds very sad. I guess it is. And here I am today, having the most trouble leaving the house. Just the idea of having to leave for work tomorrow is exhausting.

I had a nice day considering. I planted an herb garden and made banana bread and read half a book and went food shopping (horrid) and cleaned the bathroom and kitchen and fixed the backed up drain and did the laundry and that sounds like a lot but it's not enough to stop me thinking about it.

I'm thinking about taking more days at another tattoo shop because I know I'll be too busy to think, and thinking is especially painful right now.

I just practiced telling myself that my body is mine. "This is my body, this body is mine," I kept saying to myself over and over in my mind. This body that was violated. The horror and disgust of penetration was overwhelming to me as a young child, and it is again now. I remember sitting in class (first and second grade) horrified and terrified that the penises of the boys in the class would escape from them and crawl up my shorts and inside me like vicious little worms. I would have nightmares about them bursting out from the walls like in Poltergeist and flying at my head.

I think I probably imagined them disembodied like that to protect myself from the terrible reality of incest. But in my recent ayahuasca experience he was made whole again like a sinister, undead Horus. I am Isis, I made him whole with my mystic power. It was necessary to do it, but it's hard to think about now.

The victory of separating his residue from my experiences with other people is tempered by the wholeness of my knowledge. I want to be free, and the cost of freedom is the awful truth ....

I suppose truth does set free. But not many people know what free is. I'm glad to come closer and closer to existing in a state of non-resistance to reality. I don't think there's any going back from these kinds of revelations, not for people like me anyway. I just hope I can find a way to weather the truth well enough. There's a lot of good in the world, and

I've been looking for it, trying to tune my antenna to positive aspects of reality so that I can feed myself with those positive things like I used to with the negative. It's a funny process. I have a long way to go.

Despite the major revelation of Pony's early experience certain residual aspects related to her early trauma endured. Sex was still a generally dissociative event to get through, people were still difficult to take in anything more than small doses, and she preferred her own company most of the time. Pony was adamant about letting me know that the internal sense of dread and hopelessness was not a singularly triggered experience, rather, it was chronically omnipresent. Although she made rapid strides in her development as a tattoo artist it was difficult to remain in any one shop for very long. Her tolerance for being hassled had diminished now more than ever. Whenever she was sexually provoked or exploited in any manner, particularly as a woman in a strongly paternalistic profession, she moved to another shop. It was in this state of continuous unease and distress that she decided to leave New York with her tattoo mentor E, now boyfriend, in a customized van for a road trip around the United States. They would visit tattoo shops around the country as guest artists, paint trains at night, and come to know each other free of outside interference from their New York colleagues. (Pony: *The part of Jersey where I grew up is crisscrossed with rail lines. There's a pinch point that funnels down through the Ramapo mountains, connecting upstate with the ports of Hudson County. I was constantly in the care of extended family in the early years when my father was junked up and my mother working all the time, and as I would wait up late at night hoping for one of them to return, I would hear the train whistles. I knew that they could carry me away to somewhere new. There's autoracks and grainers and heaps of intermodals all moving lumber and steel and salt and paper and I wanted to move with them. I put my name on them and I am carried away, as far as Albuquerque and Portland and Mexico City and New Orleans and –*) Finally, Pony would have a chance to recapture an uncomplicated intimacy with this man who bore a strong resemblance to her lost uncle.

During the months that Pony was on the road we had intermittent communication by email. These (edited) e-mail letters chronicled the internal reflection of her trajectory simultaneously through both the country and the relationship, an autoethnography of sorts:

[My uncle] is the A-bomb as far back as I can trace, but I know there was one before him, and one before that one too. I don't know that I'll ever find out what happened and why to make them all this way. The possibility of knowing is the one thing that makes me wish he was still alive.

I want to cut out the part of me that misses the niceties of him. I think that as I digest the idea that he was wrong and I was innocent, I will do that.

... I'm finding it a lot easier to breathe out here in the midwest.

When my uncle died, it was chaos at home. A week or so later my parents split up. Everything fell apart. I was so confused about my own feelings. I was so numb at my uncle's funeral. We stayed in the house where he raped me and I had nightmares and terrifying daytime visions of a skeletal version of him – it was a figure like a holocaust victim but with his same hair and nose and mustache, and it snuck around the house laughing about how no one but me could see it. I would see it in the corner of my eye and be too afraid to turn my head toward it, because I knew I would see it plainly and no one else would, and that would mean I was crazy. It would stand over me as I lay awake in the pull out bed with my mother. I could hear my mother and my grandmother snoring, and I knew he knew they were asleep.

I always had social problems, even before he died. I was a biter in kindergarten. I was so stilted and outcast and strange in first grade that my teacher got the guidance counselor to meet with me every week. I kept struggling with social interaction and school work until fourth grade, when my uncle died. For some reason, as soon as that happened I got very focused and went from Bs and Cs to straight As.

There was a popular girl on my bus that year and I was sure she was saying bad things about me. I don't know if she was or not but I read contempt on her face when she looked at me. One day I saw her look at me and then whisper to the girl next to her and so I reached out and choked her, not very hard because I was so afraid of actually hurting her but hard enough to leave a mark.

I got detention over recess for one day. The principal knew my situation and was pretty understanding. I was glad for it to be over. But when I got back to class, my teacher Mr. E told everyone how I was in the principal's office because I did something bad and everyone oooh'd and pointed and laughed. I think I wrote him four different letters asking him to explain why he humiliated me like that. I asked him what I did to deserve extra punishment. I never gave him the letters.

Then there were band teachers and math teachers and history teachers. It started as me wanting to be good, to impress them. Then it would get weird somehow and I would be afraid and I wanted to run away. Later I started to feel that I wanted to kill them. I don't think that really solidified until I started taking voice lessons. I had that feeling toward any teacher who touched me, and you know how much touching there is in lesson. I had a math teacher who acted like he thought I was an idiot and a fuck up (I was a B-C student in core classes in high school and skipped class a lot), but one day it was cold and I was wearing a t-shirt and shivering because I'm always cold and he came around without saying anything and put his jacket on me. I guess he thought he was being kind. I still get angry when I think of him. Then there was that therapist who texted about how beautiful and smart and special I was. I had to drive by his office every time I gave a piano lesson to one of my students in Ramsey and I had so many fantasies of setting the building on fire.

When I was about 13 I kicked my mother in the jaw full force because she was tickling me. That was a recent sort of argument between me and E. I can't really call it an argument. But certain types of guys love to tickle full grown adult women (I will never understand the appeal). He used to do it all the time, and one time I told him not to. And then the next time I told him more seriously. And then some time passed but then I had to tell him again. And the last time I freaked out and had to lay it out for him that he can't tickle me because it will literally transport me through space and time back to a moment of extreme fear and discomfort.

But he was disappointed. That he couldn't tickle me anymore. The way it worked with [previous boyfriend], I think, was that tickling was a proxy for violence. Maybe it is for E too, one of the few ways he could vent his frustration at me. Never getting away from one another, living and working together in the same small space, navigating lots of complicated social and personal issues, me dealing with the results of my abuse and leaning on him for that. I understand the desire for violence by proxy. Maybe it's a healthy way for healthy people to get frustrations out and also bond at the same time, but I am not healthy like that.

Just like all the outings in hollywood, there are starting to be outings in tattooing for serial abusers and rapists. I'm glad that things are changing, in a detached way the part of me that's been flashed and peeped at and inappropriately touched and taken advantage of is glad. But at the same time I can't help but feel like all of society's sudden outrage has nothing at all to do with me. Rape is outrageous, but incest is truly disgusting.

I think Freud was wrong. I think most of the women he talked to probably were abused by their fathers and grandfathers and uncles. He couldn't bear to think it was true, and now I have penis envy. But he's wrong and it's as fucking ubiquitous as he should have thought. But thanks to him and all the rest it's fucking invisible too, and when you grapple with it everyone wants to see you as a miserable failure, because that's easier for them than having to live in a world where violent incest is as mundane as milk.

I have made the mistake of believing I am a miserable failure. I make it all the time. I'm crazy and lazy and paranoid and unable to hack life, unwilling to go outside most days and triggered all the time by the micro abuses against women and outsiders (of which I am both) that are built into the fabric of society. So ruffled and sensitive that I can't go even a day without brushing up against some thing that drives me a little bit crazy again.

The real crazy thing is most of the time when things upset me like that my reaction is to smile. To wither away inside and smile and keep on doing whatever it is I'm expected to do with my hands all shaking and without any sense. Where is the anger now? It's easier to roll over. It's too scary not to lay down and let it happen. To be angry and to resist is to be punished even more.

The clearest memory I have of him raping me seems like it was almost in reaction to my kicking and fidgeting and trying to scream as he's putting his fingers there. I was on my back and he grabbed me by the throat and by the ankles. Maybe if I was just quiet he wouldn't have put the thing in and hurt me and it could have been like the other times.

It's hard to survive and make good choices and follow through on things because the whole world's a hazard. It's hard to have decent relationships, even simple relationships like having a neighbor or a dentist or a coffee barista. It's hard and I can't do it all the time ....

I hope you are okay too. Sorry for the novella. I've included a different kind of picture this time. The more this stuff loosens up the more I'm able to draw again. I've been doodling scenes from some of my recurring nightmares. It's pretty low-fi but it helps me [see Figures 6.5–6.8 below].

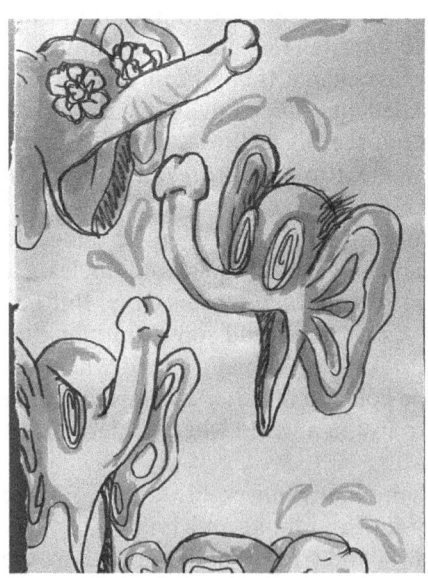

Figure 6.5 Drawing.

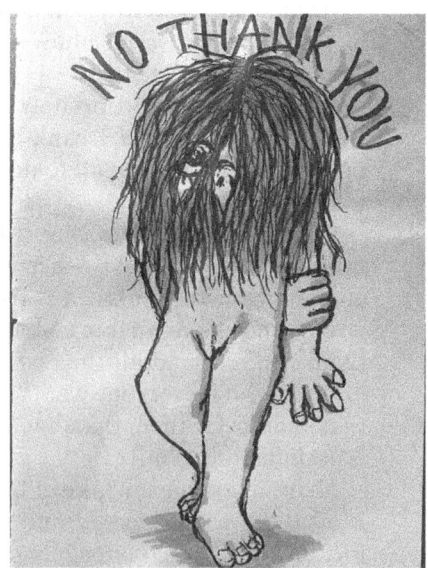

Figure 6.6 Drawing.

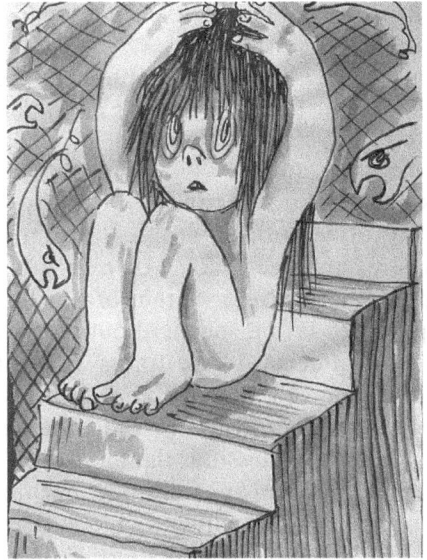

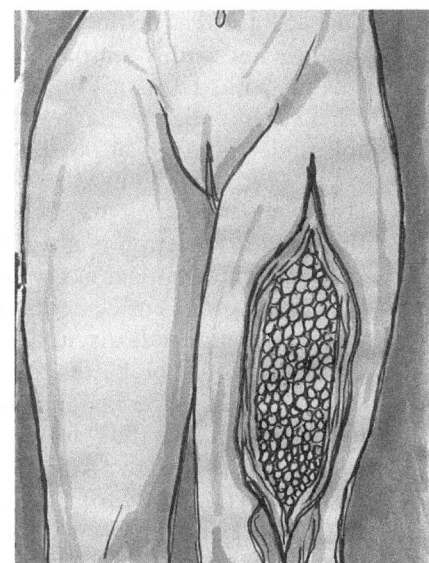

Figure 6.7 Drawing.

Figure 6.8 Drawing.

Eventually the hoped-for recovery of lost intimacy followed an all too familiar trajectory and Pony's boyfriend E gradually withdrew into himself. The emotional toll of this reenactment of abandonment proved too much and she left him out west to return home. Despite her most ardent wishes and efforts there would be no way through the recovered memory of early trauma other than to have her complete emotional response to it. But that prospect seemed truly overwhelming on a daily basis. However now, unlike when she was a small child, she had resources to face this ordeal. Principle among these resources was her habitual inclination toward visual self-representation; now incarnate with immediate, literal, and graphic relevance due to her deepening involvement in body art.

* * *

Tattoos are ubiquitous across time and space. Charles Darwin is quoted as saying, "Not one great country can be named, from the Polar region in the north to New Zealand in the south, in which the aborigines do not tattoo themselves" (quoted in Favazza 1992, 125). Moreover, the functional purposes for tattooing are as multiple and varied as the cultures in which they are found. These functions include supernatural protection, mnemonic signs, and classificatory designation. As per Pony's treatment I am focused here on the heuristic and highly speculative psychological functions of the body art of tattoos as distinct from other forms of bodily social coding like scarification and bodily mutilation.

To begin with, I began Pony's treatment with a specific notion of the body, here exemplified by Barker (1998, 10); one that admits of as many and variable understandings as possible:

> However necessary it may be to isolate the body for analytic purposes, the body in question is not a hypostatized object, still less a simple biological mechanism of given desires and needs acted on externally by controls and enticements, but a relation in a system of liaisons which are material, discursive, psychic, sexual, but without stop or center. It would be better to speak of a certain 'bodiliness' than of 'the body'. It is the instance of suturing of discourse and desire to the organism and thus fully social in its being and in its ideological valency. Rather than an extra-historical residue, invariant and mute, this body is as ready for coding and decoding, as intelligible both in its presence and its absence, as any of the more frequently recognized historical objects.

For the body that is 'ready for coding,' the tattoo may be reasonably, if not reductively, likened to an embodied screen memory. According to Freudian theory (Freud 1962b; Laplanche and Pontalis 1973), a screen memory is,

> a childhood memory characterized by both its usual sharpness and by the apparent insignificance of its content. The analysis of such memories leads back to indelible childhood experiences and to unconscious phantasies. *Like the symptom, the screen memory is a formation produced by a compromise between repressed elements and defense.*
>
> 410–411 (emphasis added)

Freud (1962a) specifically addresses the content of these 'repressed elements' in his famous early insight, directly pertaining to Pony's tattoos, where he draws a connection between sexual trauma, symptom, and mnemonic activity: "*the symptoms of hysteria are determined by certain experiences of the patient which have operated in a traumatic fashion and which are being reproduced in his psychic life in the form of mnemonic symbols*" (192–193, author's emphasis) ... [and further on] "at the bottom of every case of hysteria there are *one or more occurrences of premature sexual experience*, occurrences which belong to the earliest years of childhood" (203, author's emphasis).

In his relevant discussion of Holocaust memorials, Young (1993) also takes up the connection between trauma and memory in a way that additionally pertains to Pony's tattoo practice. We are left wondering: can the body also be viewed as a monument? Is the point of monumentalizing a body to help forget? To relieve the burden of remembering? Young suggests that "perhaps the more memory comes to rest in exteriorized forms, the less it is experienced internally" (5).

To the extent that Pony's trauma is implicated in her tattoo practice, her "[body] art is a mode of fantasy structured by the desire to escape the anxiety of influence" (Weiss 1994, 93). Moreover, as so-called compromise formations, as with all of Pony's artistic productions, her embodied images are multidetermined – they both express and protect herself. The protection or escape afforded by her tattoos is already implicit in the transposition from traumatic experience to expression. Discussing the representability of the Holocaust, Alphen (1999, author's emphasis) states,

> experience of an event or history is dependent on the terms the symbolic world offers. It needs those terms to transform living through the event into an experience of the event … The notion of experience already implies a certain degree of distance from the event; experience is the transposition of the event to the realm of the subject. Hence the experience *of* an event is already a representation of it and not the event itself.
>
> 27

This would seem to suggest a certain level of therapeutic mastery behind the composition and inscription of the images adorning Pony's body, whether in symbolic disguise or otherwise. And in fact, this function is exactly what is implied by Freud (1958) in his notion of the 'secondary elaboration' of dreams, or Lewin's (1973) idea of "syncretism," or by the later psychoanalytic ego psychologists (Nunberg 1965; Freud 1966; Hartmann 1977) in their postulated "integrative" or "synthetic" functions of the ego. In this view, composition is synonymous with soothing self-regulation or healing; a practice that makes the irrational rational. Certainly, there was evidence of all the above psychological functions present in Pony's composition, inscription, and exhibition of her tattoos. However, there were also whole realms of experience in relation to her body art that appeared affectively complex and seemed to lie beyond words. And this was all the more remarkable given how highly articulate Pony ordinarily is. When it came to speech, to talking about her body and the images on it, not to mention the action of her specific trauma, another enigmatic language, another enigmatic way of remembering predominated.

Notwithstanding my commitment to Bion's recommendation of a therapeutic stance beyond memory and desire, I sought theoretical constructs that addressed early unconscious, perhaps preverbal experience, in order to empathize with those aspects of Pony's life that lay beyond anything I had personally experienced. Throughout my career as a therapist I have self-consciously and pragmatically resorted to the theoretical constructions of other clinicians whenever I felt lost; just as one consults maps of those who had travelled before them, hoping to find familiar landmarks. Perhaps this had more to do with my own need for defensive intellectualization in the face of a horrifying experience. Nevertheless, with Pony my theoretical search was necessarily geared toward embodied knowledge. I began by considering Lewin's (1946, 88) notion of the "dream screen":

> the surface onto which a dream appears to be projected. It is the blank background, present in the dream though not necessarily seen, and the visually perceived action in ordinary manifest dream contents takes place on it or before it.

The dream screen is embodied insofar as it is based for the infant on nothing other than the mother's breast. (Pony: *Where was this place for me? Where is it in the long halls of my memory? It seems of all the fantastical shapes and figures in my internal world to be the most fleeting and dream-like.*) This insight was helpful in a derivative way toward understanding the self-soothing potential in body art production; in the same way that Pony's writing could analogously be understood as a type of automirroring. (Pony: *The mirror, the looking-glass. The gloss of a still pond, depthless and dark. For these things the light comes from without. It reflects; if I'm lucky it refracts. I had to write the very sun into existence within me for the barest glimpse of my own face. Pony, in fluorescent green, in matte Rust-Oleum's Sunburst Yellow, cans on cans, my primary color, petal-soft against concrete and steel. "Stops Rust," the can says. Halts decay.*)

Yet it seemed that the more persistently and insistently I interpreted content, the more Pony's experience was slipping away from me. In writing about her it became manifestly clear that my unthinking zeal for interpretation, so taken for granted, must have been experienced as a type of penetration, as highly invasive, and as eerily reminiscent of her earlier trauma of sexual intrusion. (Pony: *I assure you, friend, that your gentle vivisection was far preferable to the butchery of others.*) Anything resembling penetration had to be avoided. Pony could be cast into a foul mood at the idea of someone just brushing against her in the subway train on her way to see me. Grosz (1994, 79) explains,

> Just as there is a zone of sensitivity concerning the body's openings and surfaces, so too there is a zone outside the body, occupying its surrounding space, which is incorporated into the body. Intrusion into this bodily space is considered as much a violation as penetration of the body itself.

Stepping back from a depth-psychology focus I considered Pony's body art from the opposite perspective, that is, simply as her cover, her embellished skin. I consulted the work of Anzieu (1990, 2010) who infers a parallel between the cover of the body, our skin, the largest organ of our body, and a psychic 'skin ego.' The skin ego, according to Anzieu, has from the birth of the human individual a containing function that he likened to a 'skin-envelope.' (Pony: *To whom do I address these epistles, hm? That the mirror of another should dictate back to me the contents of my own skin? How terribly lonely.*) The skin, as Taylor (1997, 12) points out, also ordinarily has a "duplicitous" function: "Hide hides." Building on these conventional notions of skin as holding, enveloping, and hiding it was left for me to imagine the psychological consequences of actual sexual intercourse between an adult man and a very small child. (Pony: *And again, for having asked of you this wretched work, I'm sorry.*)

It is my belief that for Pony, early notions of inside and outside, of boundedness and containment, were severely disrupted. Thus any ensuing notion of self in relation to other, of privacy, of internal versus external, would be radically altered. And any search for an underlying code in her presentation posed the risk of irrelevance at best, further traumatization at worst.

I clung to the notion that my empathic shortcomings were not so much a lack of caring as a "failure of translation" between highly disparate experiential, psychological developmental "codes" (Laplanche 2011). And it is to this failure of translation that I attribute my provisional characterization of Pony's early world as existing in a realm of formlessness. This Bataillean (1991a) notion of formlessness is, I believe, synonymous with what Lacan describes as the Real:

> The real is 'the impossible' because it is impossible to imagine, impossible to integrate into the symbolic order, and impossible to attain in any way. It is this character of impossibility and of resistance to symbolization which lends the real it's essentially traumatic quality.
>
> Evans (1996, 160)

In fact, the role of *empathy* itself, considered by self-psychology to be a central healing force in treatment (Kohut 1984) and relying as it does on introspection, could not be taken for granted as an innocuous aid in my work with Pony. To wit: "Empathy does indeed define the *field* of our observations ... the idea itself of an inner life of man, and thus of a psychology of complex mental states, is unthinkable without our ability to know via vicarious introspection" (Kohut 1986, 306, author's emphasis). Any idea of empathy with Pony would have to be predicated on my demonstrated understanding of the challenges that come with living so exposed in a world where everyone else takes inside and outside for granted. Hence my focus on the medium by which Pony could most easily express herself – her tattoos.

Pony described the functional importance of tattooing her toes as a transformational aid for forgetting the visual image of her feet up in the air while being raped (see Figure 6.12). At other times, she directly stated the wish to reclaim her violated body through her body art, thereby redefining herself as more than a victim. These efforts to address an inner experience through re-exteriorization are addressed by Schilder (1978) who states,

> It is a new proof of the lability of the body-image that whatever comes into connection with the surface of our body is more or less incorporated into the body. [Pony: *This includes hands and mouths and fluids, fingers and lingering bruises, doesn't it? As much as it includes the things I choose, it must include those that I didn't. If I see a rival, an enemy's name on a train car, I cover it with my own. I write him out of existence as I write myself in.*] We know that many attempts are made to change the body-image. Pictures may be drawn on the skin. Tattooing changes the optic part of ourselves. [Pony: *It's beyond optics. If optics sufficed, why not a cloak? No, I had to overwrite the hidden things, the things that were until recently very nearly unseeable.*] When we paint our body we change the body-image in an objective way.
>
> 202

This important ordinary malleability of the interior versus exterior basis of body image is also attested to by Scarry (1985, 384)

> The interchange of inside and outside surfaces requires not the literal reversal of body linings but the making of what is originally interior and private into something exterior and sharable, and, conversely, the reabsorption of what is now exterior and sharable into the recesses of individual consciousness.

Both Scarry's and Schilder's ideas help illuminate Pony's experience to the extent that we can now understand how the body surface, and by extension the body image, can be manipulated to simultaneously express experience beyond (or before) verbal articulation. It also throws light on her heightened sensitivity to her surroundings. With an appreciation for the vital importance of boundaries, I reconsidered Pony's presenting problem entering treatment – her blocked creative output – as a fear regarding the potential failure of her container, containing as it did the knowledge of transgression that could kill if it were 'let out.' In her famous essay "On not being able to paint," Joanna Field (1957, 16) describes,

> I noticed that the effort needed in order to see the edges of objects as they really looked stirred a dim fear, a fear of what might happen if one let

go one's mental hold on the outline which kept everything separate and in its place; and it was similar to that fear of a wide focus of attention.

(Pony: *This recalls the persistent and claustrophobic attenuation of my senses in times of heightened anxiety. I do not see it, I refuse to see it, I am looking away. I cannot see it, and so slowly I go blind.)*

Gradually, and with extraordinary patience from Pony, I drew closer to understanding her experience. This was enabled in large part by anthropologist Michael Taussig (1992) who, writing from an ethnographic perspective that equally applies to clinical treatment, eschews depth interpretation in favor of a tactile knowledge. Regarding psychoanalytic interpretation,

> such a mode of analysis is simple-minded in its search for 'codes' and manipulative because it superimposes meaning on 'the native's point of view.' Rather, as I now understand this practice of reading, its very understanding of 'meaning' is uncongenial; its weakness lies in its assuming a contemplative individual when it should, instead, assume a distracted collective reading with a tactile eye.
>
> 147

Moreover, social anthropologist Connerton (1996) suggests that this orientation of tactility must reach into our clinical understanding of memory:

> meaning cannot be reduced to a sign which exists on a separate level outside the immediate sphere of the body's acts. Habit is a knowledge and a remembering in the hands and in the body; and in the cultivation of habit it is our body which 'understands'.
>
> 95

Pony had continuously stressed the importance of the physical pain involved in receiving a tattoo, perhaps even more than any message associated with the finished result. Lingis (1983, 22) addresses this specific aspect of body art:

> What we are dealing with is inscription. Where writing, graphics, is not inscription on clay tablets, bark, or papyrus, but in flesh and blood. Where it is not significant, not a matter of marks whose role is to signify, to efface themselves before the meaning, or ideality, or logos. For here the signs count: they hurt. Before they make sense to the reader, they give pain to the living substrate.

Lingis goes even further, extending the emphasis on the sensuous experience of body inscription to Pony's other favored form of artistic expression – graffiti art:

> It belongs to the nature of graffiti not to pay heed to borders, to spread right over obstacles, to make walls of different angles, doors, openings, all the support of one inscription that supports itself. The inscription extends the erotogenic surface ... We say that these incisions, these welts and scars, these graphics, are not signs, they are intensive points. They do not refer to intentions in an inner individual psychic depth, not to meanings and concepts in some transcendent beyond. They reverberate one another.
>
> 37

(Pony: *Anyone who studies graffiti knows this to be true. The name alone is not enough. The name in context is everything. To write in this furtive, antisocial way is to touch through the medium of the wall. It's the soothing of a deep loneliness. The name alone is meaningless. The name in context has shape, has style. Nothing is more lonely than a single name on a water tower, in a cornfield in the daytime ...*)

Pony's praxis of tattooing was of twofold sensuous significance. As the recipient, the reenactment of trauma through the painful inscription was invariably followed by what Pony described as a state of euphoria. As the providing tattoo artist, Pony described her exquisite care for the emotional and physiological experience of her clients who handled their pain in a variety of ways. Certainly this latter scenario conforms to a relational experience close to projective identification. Yet any attempt to focus on reenactment or significance that departed from the sensuality of her body practices threatened to undermine empathy as I now understood it.

Rather than continuing my search "inside" Pony's psychology for the key that decodes her increasingly self-designed body, I began searching for the "outer" cultural context, the "ecological niche" if you will, that would most compatibly reverberate with her aesthetically re-exteriorized body (see Hacking 1998, 1). Lingis's (1983) insightful observations on bodily inscription and its place in the life of the individual and society were made possible by his immersion in the Maasai culture of Africa, courtesy of Kenya-born photographer Mirella Ricciardi (1974). In a similar vein, I considered Pony's preference for the company of animals; her facility with nonverbal modes of communication (whether that be through her study of music or her work tutoring autistic children); and her lifelong devotion to artistic representation through various media, particularly of animals and human/animal hybrids. Added to this was Pony's comfort in embryonic-like spaces at both home and work as derivative of her keen awareness of inside versus outside. Lastly, I conjectured that her extremely early exposure to sexual behavior with an adult, occurring as it did before she developed the cognitive ability to process it, predisposed her to be extraordinarily attuned to the animality of human sexual interaction – "Only in the most extreme moments is animality confronted" (Pawlett 2016, 16). (Pony: *If this is true for others, I'm glad for them. No, for me such closeness is bestial, a riot of scents and textures and twisted expressions, a study in the ways in which men depart themselves when they enter into me. Horrible, horrible. It isn't even a truth laid bare. It's a lateral slide, a departure from a mode and by that departure, an excuse: to be animal, as they understand it. To abandon 'reason,' as they understand it. And I, who retain my state still the same, am the one who appears strange. Alluring, but strange. But it's you who are strange, baffled by your own attachment to rationality [and needing that lateral release because of it] and easily tricked by your own selves. I am not so easily tricked. There's no joy you could give me as you are then. I don't share your hunger. What could your body offer me that isn't eclipsed tenfold by the animal world? I don't want you inside me, and so. A tiger is more elegant, a horse more pleasing to touch, even soaked in the sweat of exertion. The myopic eyes of a cow see me more clearly than you do then. Enough.*) The sum impression of all these and more features of our work intuitively led me to adopt the idea of the prehistoric cave, particularly like those at Lascaux that featured Neolithic cave painting, along with Georges Bataille's interpretation of them, as the analogous, heuristic context within/ against which Pony's experience might be comprehended.

* * *

Leroi-Gourhan (1993) insists that Neolithic inhabitants lived commonly in huts thus ordinarily only resorting to the caves for purposes beyond simple survival. According to the archaeological excavation of the Chauvet cave, the cave was not inhabited, showed signs of fire for lighting but no hearths for cooking, and were most likely visited intermittently by bears (Chauvet, Deschamps, and Hillaire 1996). Lewis-Williams (2002) proposes a relationship between the shape of the caves and the cosmologies of their visitors as well as between the topographies of the caves and their visitors' social structure. He goes on further to suggest that the nervous system of Neolithic peoples predisposed them to easily access altered states of consciousness as evidenced in the nearly universal appearance of similarities in cave use, and particularly, their cave art. Thus, there is the suggestion of continuity between cave structure, human social life, and human consciousness. (Pony: *True enough; I am the cave, into which you come to experience another state. Enough.*)

Bataille imagines "that humans may have been motivated to make their own markings on cave walls after observing scratches made by bears" (Richman 2018, 165). To explain what appears to be a pattern of mimetic identification between hominids and animals in both ritual activity and cave paintings Clottes and Lewis-Williams (1998) have invoked the figure of the shaman. However there may be no need to postulate a specialist, such as a shaman, to explain this strangely expressed affinity. Rather, the mimetic faculty may be considered a fundamentally, perhaps quintessentially human trait of any and all cave visitors/artists, indeed of most, if not all, Neolithic protohumans. Benjamin (1999) implies as much:

> Nature produces similarities, one need only think of mimicry. The highest capacity for producing similarities, however, is man's. His gift for seeing similarity is nothing but a rudiment of the once powerful compulsion to become similar and to behave mimetically. There is perhaps not a single one of his higher functions in which the mimetic faculty does not play a decisive role ... clearly the perceptual world of modern man contains only minimal residues of the magical correspondences and analogies that were familiar to ancient peoples. The question is whether we are concerned with the decay of this faculty or with its transformation.
>
> 720–721

In his modern ethnographic research, Lewis-Williams (1992) encounters Kung San bushmen of the Kalahari moving in and out of trance states and again wonders: are they shamans? Lewis-Williams is engaging here in precisely the same activity as myself: he is resorting to a known cultural form to try and make sense of an experience that ultimately lies beyond him. Do the bushmen and Neolithic cave visitors fulfill that specialty role as technicians of the sacred (Eliade 1974)? Or is it as Jaynes (1982) suggests that a different consciousness prevailed in prehistory for all, a consciousness alternative and unrecognizable to our modern selves? Perhaps a once ubiquitous consciousness that is available today only through regression brought on by extreme deprivation, pain, sickness, and other forms of traumatic excess as well as entheogenic substances?

The combination of foregoing archaeological clues, notwithstanding their highly speculative nature, serve as a helpful entry into Bataille's understanding of the painted caves. The altered state of consciousness, one that may have been characterized by a primacy of tactile awareness and knowledge; the contiguous residence with animal neighbors; and their mimetic representation on cave walls; would all suggest an earlier state of hominid continuity with animals that is so important in Bataille's thought.

According to Bataille, any primitive type of human social arrangement that involves classification, kinship, designation, taboos, prohibitions, and rules betrays a Neolithic preoccupation with distinguishing themselves from animals. This would seem to accord with Lacan who asserts that the crucial developmental entry of the infant into the social world of humans is contingent on the rule of "Non" from the father. Yet Bataille will further argue that the rise of the social world itself was not attributable to social laws, that its impetus was in play – play as originally captured through form and content in the paintings of the caves. Bataille states (1955, 27, author's emphases),

> At the outset art was primarily a game. In a major sense it still is. It is play; while tool-making is primarily work. To establish the meaning of Lascaux (by which I mean the epoch of which Lascaux is the materialization) is to perceive the shift from the world of work to the world of play; or the transition from *Homo faber* to *Homo sapiens*: from the roughhewn to the finished human being.

The equation of play and art is by no means unique to Bataille (see Huizinga 1955), nor is the equation between play and the sacred (see Caillois 2001). What distinguishes Bataille (1992b) is the assertion that this early sacred play was erotic in nature and, insofar as the cave hominids remained acutely aware of their animal origins, was strongly connected to their dawning, distinctive awareness of separation, loss, and death.

For Bataille, the cave represents the point of separation where the human emerges quite literally in form through the cave paintings as distinct from other animals. The cave is thus the locus for the emergence of form from what Bataille would identify as formlessness. It is sacred not only for its devotion to play over production for survival; but more importantly, its sacred character derives from its devotion to the growing ambivalent regard for their own animality in relation to their animal neighbors. The cave paintings, themselves being compromise formations between reverence and repulsion, are a tribute to the emergence of a distinctly human reality; one that entails non-productive consciousness of loss, separateness, death, and erotic play. And as discussed earlier with regard to Pony's tattoos, the cave painters derived benefit from the "secondary elaboration" of their art. "The representation of animals is a sacred activity to the extent that they embody the forces of life and death which can be dominated more readily within the cave than outside it" (Ungar 1990, 256).

The paintings depict the construction of a tenuous reality that requires both an acknowledgement and a repudiation of our own animality and is thus considered sacred by Bataille. Pawlett (2016, 5) states,

> for Bataille there is a more fundamental terror: a terror of formlessness and a failure of language to confront human immanence or 'continuity' in the world. Only that restricted, artificial construct 'reality' has form,

and reality has form because it denies, refuses, rejects, or destroys all instances of formlessness.

Bataille (1991b)

will identify the cave paintings as only the beginning foundation of a set of prohibitions and restrictions on which a distinctive and social human reality develops: "The incest prohibition is one of the effects of the repugnance felt for his condition by the animal that became human. The forms of animality were excluded from a bright world which signified humanity" (61–62). (Bataille is here expanding on Lévi-Strauss (1969, 10) who remarks on the centrality of the incest taboo: "Few social prescriptions in our society have so kept that aura of respectful fear which clings to sacred objects.") The distinct category of "human" is acquired at a price; there is an inherent, internal conflict on which he/she exists, the internally repressed animal will forever haunt from within. Bataille (1992a) warns, "The definition of the animal as a thing has become a human given. The animal has lost its status as man's fellow creature, and man, perceiving the animal in himself, regards it as a defect" (39). (Pony: *I am not so easily tricked.*)

On account of her early trauma of sexual incest, Pony felt incomplete as a human. She could easily assimilate into an anime landscape for hours as a child, or imagine herself transported to a mythical, mystical world of her own making. However, more than anything else her affinity for animals was persistent and enduring; as evidenced both with her lifelong pet companions and in the form of the guardian spirit animals that she encountered during her ayahuasca sessions. This kinship she felt with animals was expressed through drawings from early childhood and is now inscribed graphically over her entire body. Although she is covered from head to toe with tattoos today, she has selected five specific tattoo images to exhibit for this project. Their location on her body is identified on a topographic map of her own construction, commonly used in her profession, displaying the location of these specific tattoos on the front and back of her body (see Figure 6.9).

This seemingly random selection of images out of dozens follows an idiosyncratic, if not emotional, logic which is elaborated below. The format of a topographic map followed by an individual itemization of its specific contents is suggested by Leroi-Gourhan's (1967) catalogue of numerous European prehistoric caves.

Tattoo A (see Figure 6.10) is an exact duplicate of the same tattoo that her Uncle C wore on the outside of his upper right arm. The position of this image on the inside of Pony's upper right arm suggests that it is both private (somewhat concealed) and deeply personal (literally close to her heart). More than any other of her tattoos, this image embodies the conjectured mentality of the cave artists insofar as it establishes a mimetic identification with another (animal/human) being that consists of both attraction and

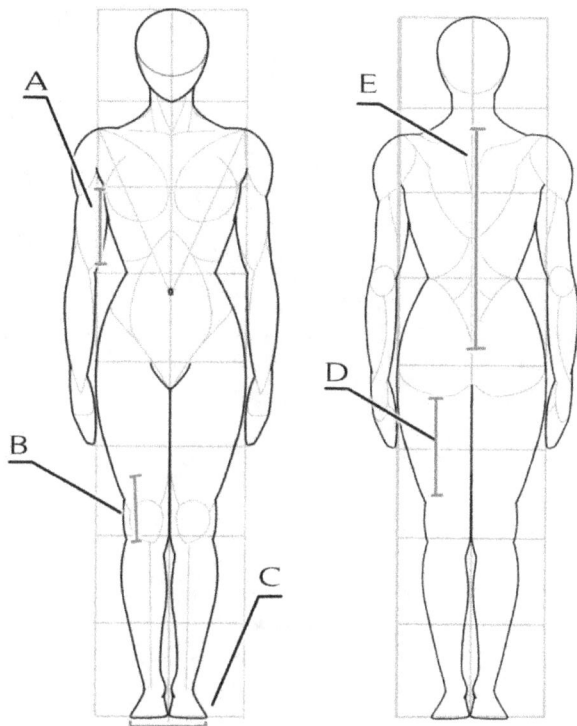

Figure 6.9 Pony's tattoo topography.

repulsion. It memorializes Pony's primordial experience of sex, violence, and death all introduced to her by her uncle. (Pony: *Since the day as a young child I first saw a relief of the god Set [god of chaos and sex and violence and strangeness, of otherness and foreignness] I have been drawn to His image. No thing is evil except uncreative destruction, which the ancient Egyptians personified in the serpent Ap[ep]. Of all the gods, only Set is strong enough to vanquish the serpent each night. I feel that chaos and uncreative destruction all worked through Uncle C in those moments we were together. He sought to annihilate me exactly as he was crossing into the generative moment of orgasm [after all, the ancient Egyptians depict the moment of universal creation as an orgasm ex nihilo; out of nothing came not the word, but the seed]. He showed me the face of annihilation, but also the face of the vital chaos that is annihilation's undoing. This mark is a symbol of devotion to that chaos which is the buffer between harmony [Ma'at] and annihilation, done in the god's favorite color, red. I am aligned with the same chaos that gave Uncle C his power, it's in*

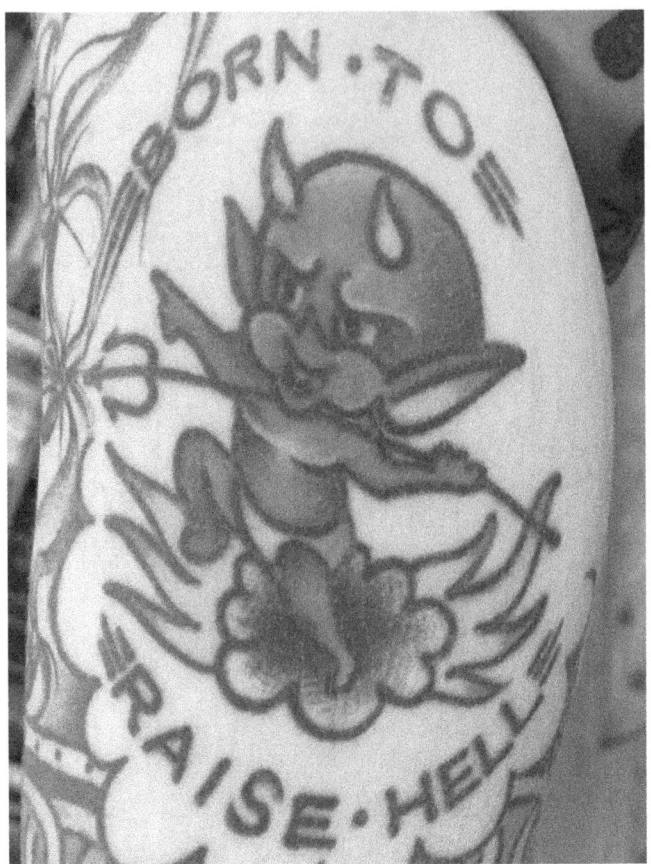

Figure 6.10 Tattoo A.

our blood, we are in and of it together. I wear Set's rabbit's ears in my dreams and I hold His scepter in my dreams. The moment of almost-destruction is the moment of my birth, and the god of chaos is my father and my lover all at once. It's only through chaos that we're delivered from the serpent's jaws to safety, and so: this reminder.) It is his power removed and taken for herself. And in taking this from him, it is a reminder that potentially enables her to forget.

Tattoo B (see Figure 6.11), the image of an eye on Pony's knee, is notable for two reasons. First, she inscribed this tattoo on her body herself; second, the eye image appears over her body more than any other. The eye image, as discussed earlier in reference to all of Pony's images, is multidetermined. That is, it both offers supernatural protection and threatens danger (see Elworthy 1895, for the classic compendium of examples from around the world since antiquity; and Spooner (1976), among many others, who attests

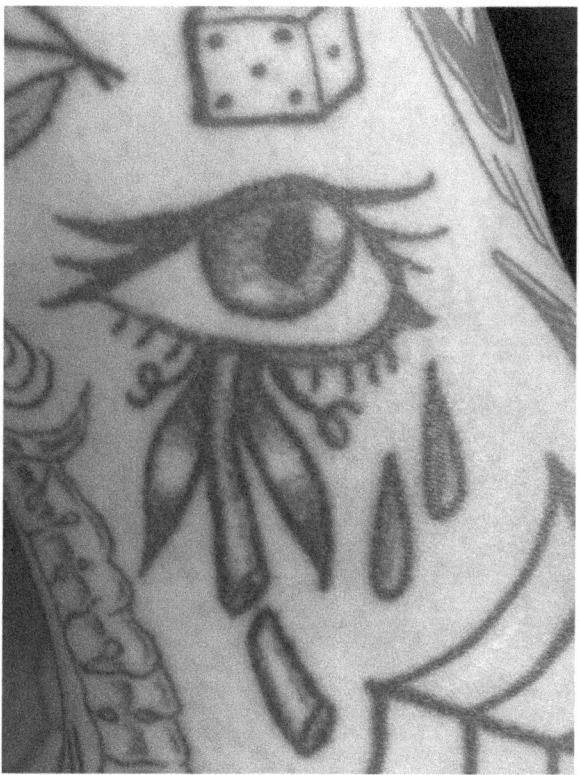

Figure 6.11 Tattoo B.

to the "defensive" nature of the eye tattoo). (Pony: *The sun god sends his daughters, his eyes, to exact his revenge. His daughters, whose righteous anger is power. An old myth says that all humans are the tears of the sun god. And those of us who bear righteous anger are both the eye and the tears. I did this tattoo when I was very very sad.*) Regarding graphic eye symbols, "The wearer is even more protected if it be written on some part of the wearer, which seems to suggest that the figures and signs which men had tattooed on their bodies carried with them some magical protection" (Budge 1992, 43). For the purpose of enhanced protection, Pony is planning to add yet another eye behind her thereby extending her "view."

As mentioned above, Tattoo C (see Figure 6.12) was inscribed for the specific purpose of altering Pony's perception of her feet and, by extension, the visceral association to her unadorned feet that she viewed while being sexually assaulted as a child. In that respect the feet tattoos are protective as an anti-mnemonic device. To the extent that body image, memory, and

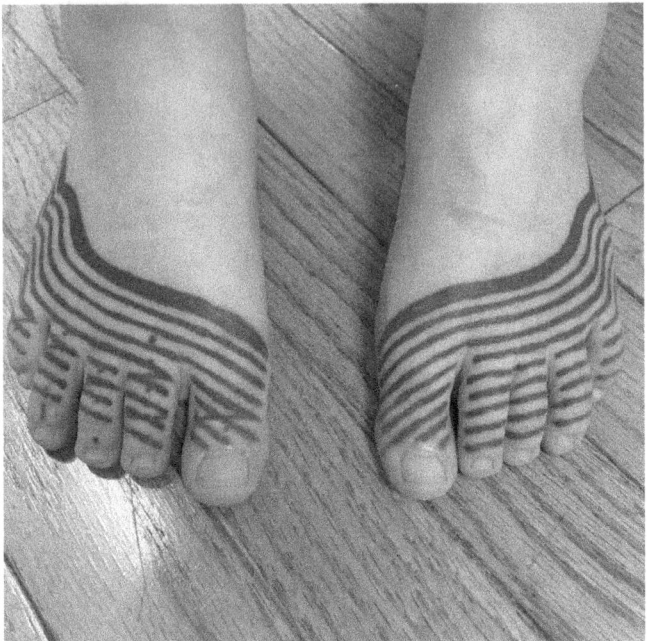

Figure 6.12 Tattoo C.

emotional experience are together impacted through the re-exteriorization of the body covering, Pony seeks here to overlay and over-write her trauma. And to the extent that the inscription of the ink into her feet hurt, she is also over-writing the pain of premature intercourse with a different pain of her own choosing. The chosen embodied form now can preempt the image of her feet whose association was to the emotional experience of trauma. (Pony: *It has become just a little bit easier to look at my own body. It has not become any easier to be observed. It's all a little cipher between me and all eyes, including my own. I dare you to decode, I dare myself to decode. I welcome a misreading; in being misread, I am shielded.*)

Tattoo D (see Figure 6.13) is an image of a snake, located on the back of her left thigh. The snake is a potent symbol for Pony since childhood and was importantly encountered during one of her ayahuasca sessions. The snake is one of at least three guardian animals that Pony relies on for protection and guidance. (Pony: *How nice to be a rattlesnake, to have a noisy little tail to tell people away, and two fangs for the ones that don't listen. The snake is like a women because his knowledge and his power is maligned in this half of history. What a shame.*)

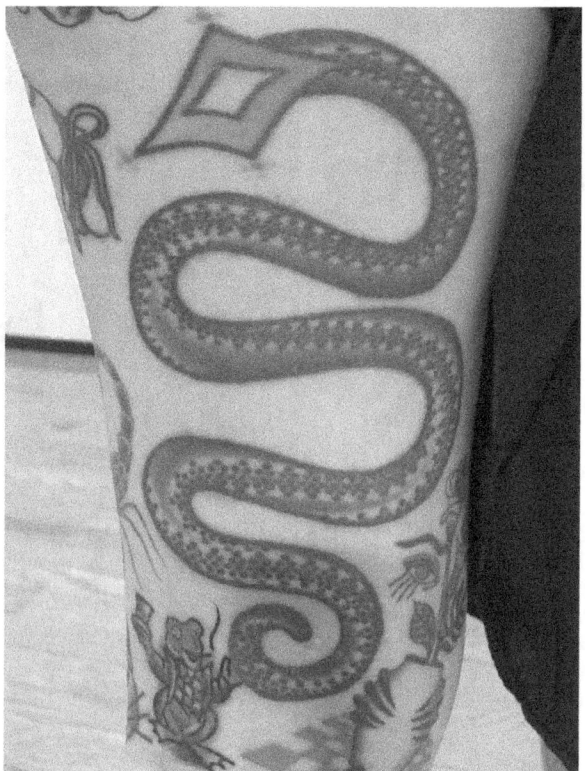

Figure 6.13 Tattoo D.

Tattoo E (see Figure 6.14) is of a large black jaguar and extends over Pony's whole back from her hips to her shoulders. Pony encountered this large black jaguar during an ayahuasca session during which she experienced it, however fearfully, as a protector and a guardian spirit animal. The curandeiro who led Pony's ayahuasca sessions informed her that it was known in Tupi-Guaraní as Otorongo and would be an invaluable guide and protector for her. The inscription of the jaguar on her body is intended to both memorialize this important encounter and enshrine the protection it offered. (Pony: *The jaguar is the savior; the jaguar is me.*)

* * *

In the same way Pony developed a means to over-write her history with her body art, she also found a way to overwrite a vulnerable, socially marginalized childhood through her identification with the figure of the

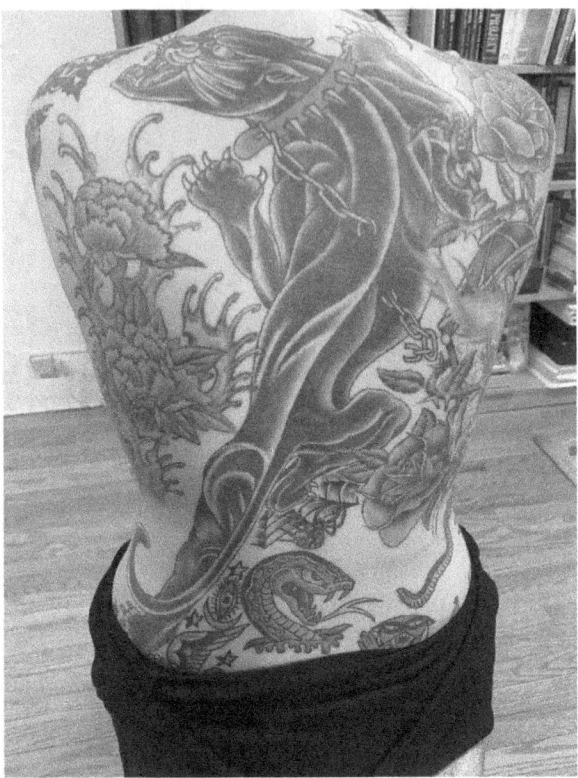

Figure 6.14 Tattoo E.

shaman. Beyond her direct experience with a self-identified shaman during her ayahuasca experiences, her rapport with animals and her turning to them for protection are established tenets of shamanism in the anthropological literature (Tedlock and Tedlock 1975; Guss 1985; Halifax 1991). As discussed earlier with Lewis-Williams, the idea of the shaman appeals to the Western imagination being an understandable response to the estrangement from our own animality as discussed by Bataille. For Pony, adopting the concept of shamanism to give form to her experience made sense given that her vulnerability necessitated a guardian or protector and "shamanism ... is practically everywhere in some fashion or in some aspect built around the vision-guardian spirit complex" (Benedict 1923, 67). In the context of her history shamanism could provide Pony with the language that rationalized her need, both retrospectively and today.

As I followed Pony's engagement with shamanism, I became increasingly interested in ways to move beyond the limits of the psychotherapy I usually offered. I had already been aware of Lévi-Strauss's (1963) famous link between shamanism and psychoanalysis:

> The modern version of shamanistic technique called psychoanalysis thus derives its specific characteristics from the fact that in industrial civilization there is no longer any room for mythical time, except with man himself. From this observation, psychoanalysis can draw confirmation of its validity, as well as hope of strengthening its theoretical foundations and understanding better the reasons for its effectiveness, by comparing its methods and goals with that of its precursors, the shamans and the sorcerers.
>
> 204

However, Grof (1988), appropriating the shamanic metaphor, goes even further in promoting an expanded exploration of "transpersonal" experience:

> As long as the process of experiential therapy focuses on the biographical level, the results are generally rather limited, unless the material that is confronted involves unfinished gestalts of serious physical traumas. The immediate and long-term results become much more dramatic when the self-exploration deepens and involves sequences of birth and death. The importance of these deeper experiences, so well-known to our shamanic ancestors, has heretofore largely escaped the notice of Western verbal psychotherapists...where the deep roots of the problem reach into the transpersonal domain, final resolution will not be reached until the client allows himself or herself to confront the specific type of transpersonal experience with which it is connected. It can be an identification with an animal form, an archetypal or mythological sequence ....
>
> 174

Ultimately, the actual historical and dynamic practice of shamanism proved less important to me than the idea of it that offers our imagination – whether the refuge for our imagination be on a body, in a cave, or in a session – the freedom to playfully reflect and form, deform, reform, and inform our experience. And so it was in the spirit of play that I asked Pony to join me in a project that would give form to our experience. Her heroic courage, her adventurous spirit, and her generous heart are all expressed here; in her words, her photos, and her art – not least of which is the drawing of an enchanted pigeon that she presented to me as a gift (see Figure 6.15). (Pony: *Truth is hidden in plain sight, in the things we dismiss out of habit. Who decides which doves are good and which are revolting and why? Who exalts only one kind of dove, and why not the other?*)

This magical bird now joins all the images herein: the animals, people, hybrid creatures, glyphs, and watchful eye. Not to be merely interpreted for,

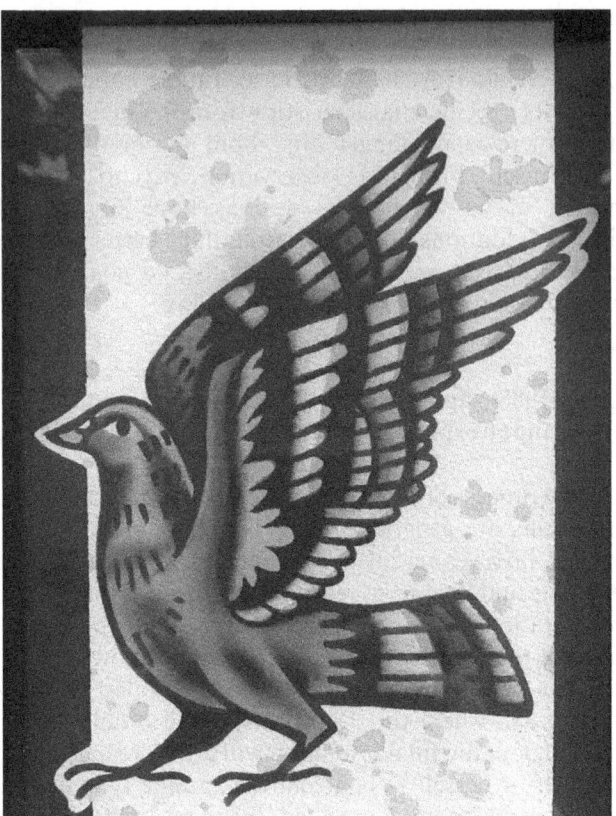

Figure 6.15 Pony's enchanted pigeon.

rather, "they reverberate one another." After all, their greatest magic might lie in their combined power to deliver you from an unimaginable experience of traumatic formlessness. Thank you, Pony, for allowing me to meet, interact, and be changed by this community of your own creation. (Pony: *And thank you, my friend. Without you none of us would be here. Like the deer that hides his malady from those around him till the wolf's jaws close, I had lain hobbled and bleeding for years. Years! The world as it was when we met had grown small and dark and hopeless. But then you peeked beneath the shroud of my unhappiness and saw the sad creature beneath. It banished my terrible loneliness, to be seen. What a shock, what dread. What a horrible exercise it was to expose you to such things. And to be thanked for doing it. Ridiculous, truly, I laugh. I laugh now with my whole body and I smile with my whole face and that wasn't always true, you know. You sat with us in the darkness with no shield. You reached into the furnace with your own bare hands to drag us out. To remind us of the world beyond. How far we've come since then! Dread has become gladness, and I hope again. I dream again. Thank you. Thank you.*)

But now the stark dignity of
entrance – Still, the profound change
Has come upon them: rooted, they
grip down and begin to awaken

William Carlos Williams (1938)

Bibliography

Alphen, Ernst Van. "Symptoms of Discursivity: Experience, Memory, Trauma." In *Acts of Memory: Cultural Recall in the Present*, 24–38. Edited by Mieke Bal, Jonathan Crewe, and Leo Spitzer. Hanover, NH: University Press of New England, 1999.

Anzieu, Didier. *A Skin for Thought: Interviews with Gilbert Tarrab on Psychology and Psychoanalysis*. Translated by Daphne Nash Briggs. New York: Karnac Books, 1990.

Anzieu, Didier. "Functions of the Skin Ego." In *Reading French Psychoanalysis*, 477–495. Edited by Dana Birksted-Breen, Sara Flanders, and Alain Gibeault. New York: Routledge, 2010/1985.

Artaud, Antonin. "The Body is the Body." In *Semiotext(e)*, 59. Translated by Roger McKeon. Vol. II (3), 1977/1947.

Barker, Francis. *The Tremulous Private Body: Essays on Subjectivism*. Ann Arbor, MI: University of Michigan Press, 1998.

Bataille, Georges. *Lascaux or the Birth of Art: Prehistoric Painting*. Translated by Austryne Wainhouse. New York: Skira Publishers, 1955.

Bataille, Georges. "Formless." In *Visions of Excess Selected Writings, 1927–1939*, 31. Edited and translated by Allan Stoekl. Minneapolis, MN: University of Minnesota Press, 1991a/1929.

Bataille, Georges. *The Accursed Share: An Essay on General Economy, Vols II and III*. Translated by Robert Hurley. New York: Zone Books, 1991b.

Bataille, Georges. *Theory of Religion*. Translated by Robert Hurley. New York: Zone Books, 1992a.

Bataille, Georges. *The Tears of Eros*. Translated by Peter Connor. San Francisco, CA: City Lights Books, 1992b.

Benedict, Ruth Fulton. *The Concept of the Guardian Spirit in North America*. Menasha, WI: Collegiate Press, 1923.

Benjamin, Walter. "On the Mimetic Faculty." In *Walter Benjamin, Selected Writings, Vol. 2*, 720–722. Edited by Michael W. Jennings, Howard Eiland, and Gary Smith. Translated by Rodney Livingstone. Cambridge, MA: Belknap Press, 1999/1933.

Bion, Wilfred. "Notes on Memory and Desire." In *Classics in Psychoanalytic Technique*, 259–260. Edited by Robert Langs. New York: Jason Aronson, 1981.

Breuer, Josef and Freud, Sigmund. "Studies in Hysteria." In *The Standard Edition of the Complete Psychological Works of Sigmund Freud, Volume II*, 1–335. Edited and translated by James Strachey. London: The Hogarth Press, 1957/1895.

Budge, Sir Wallis. *Amulets and Talismans*. New York: Carol Publishing, 1992/1930.

Caillois, Roger. *Man and the Sacred*. Translated by Meyer Barash. Chicago, IL: University of Illinois Press, 2001/1939.

Chauvet, Jean-Marie, Eliette Brunel Deschamps, and Christian Hillaire. *Dawn of Art: The Chauvet Cave, the Oldest Known Paintings in the World*. Translated by Paul G. Bahn. New York: Harry N. Abrams Publishers, 1996.

Clottes, Jean and David Lewis-Williams. *The Shamans of Prehistory: Trance and Magic in the Painted Caves*. Translated by Sophie Hawkes. New York: Harry N. Abrams Publishers, 1998.

Cixous, Helene and Catherine Clement. *The Newly Born Woman*. Translated by Betsy Wing. Minneapolis, MN: University of Minnesota Press, 1986.

Connerton, Paul. *How Societies Remember*. New York: Cambridge University Press, 1996.

Crews, Frederick. *The Memory Wars: Freud's Legacy in Dispute*. New York: New York Review Book, 1995.

Eliade, Mircea. *Shamanism: Archaic Techniques of Ecstasy*. Translated by Willard R. Trask. Princeton, NJ: Princeton University Press, 1974.

Elworthy, Frederick Thomas. *The Evil Eye: An Account of This Ancient and Widespread Superstition*. London: John Murray, Albemarle Street, 1895.

Evans, Dylan. *An Introductory Dictionary of Lacanian Psychoanalysis*. New York: Routledge, 1996.

Favazza, Armando R. *Bodies under Siege: Self-mutilation in Culture and Society*. Baltimore, MD: Johns Hopkins University Press, 1992.

Ferenczi, Sandor. "Confusion of Tongues between Adults and the Child: The Language of Tenderness and of Passion." In *Final Contributions to the Problems and Methods of Psychoanalysis*, 156–167. Edited by Michael Balint. Translated by Eric Mosbacher. New York: Brunner/Mazel Publishers, 1980/1933.

Field, Joanna. *On Not Being Able to Paint, 2nd Edition*. London: Heinemann, 1957.

Freud, Sigmund. "The Interpretation of Dreams (Second Part)." In *The Standard Edition of the Complete Psychological Works of Sigmund Freud, Volume V*, 339–627. Edited and translated by James Strachey. London: The Hogarth Press, 1958/1900.

Freud, Sigmund. "Recommendations to Physicians Practicing Psychoanalysis." In *The Standard Edition of the Complete Psychological Works of Sigmund Freud, Volume XII*, 109–120. Edited and translated by James Strachey. London: The Hogarth Press, 1958c/1912.

Freud, Sigmund. "Creative Writers and Day-dreaming." In *The Standard Edition of the Complete Psychological Works of Sigmund Freud, Volume IX*, 141–153. Edited and translated by James Strachey. London: The Hogarth Press, 1959/1908.

Freud, Sigmund. "The Aetiology of Hysteria." In *The Standard Edition of the Complete Psychological Works of Sigmund Freud, Volume III*, 189–224. Edited and translated by James Strachey. London: The Hogarth Press, 1962a/1896.

Freud, Sigmund. "Screen Memories." In *The Standard Edition of the Complete Psychological Works of Sigmund Freud, Volume III*, 301–322. Edited and translated by James Strachey. London: The Hogarth Press, 1962b/1899.

Freud, Anna. *Ego and the Mechanisms of Defense, Revised Edition*. Translated by Cecil Baines. New York: International Universities Press, 1966/1936.

Giordano, Joe and Monica McGoldrick. "Italian Families." In *Ethnicity and Family Therapy, 2nd Edition*, 567–582. Edited by Monica McGoldrick, Joe Giordano, and John K. Pearce. New York: Guilford Press, 1996.

Grof, Stanislav. "The Shamanic Journey: Observations from Holotropic Therapy." In *Shaman's Path: Healing, Personal Growth, and Empowerment*, 161–176. Compiled and edited by Gary Doore. Boston, MA: Shambhala Press, 1988.

Grosz, Elizabeth. *Volatile Bodies: Toward a Corporeal Feminism*. Bloomington, IN: Indiana University Press, 1994.

Guss, David M. (ed.). *The Language of the Birds: Tales, Texts, and Poems of Interspecies Communication*. San Francisco, CA: North Point Press, 1985.

Hacking, Ian. *Mad Travelers: Reflections on the Reality of Transient Mental Illnesses*. Charlottesville, VA: University Press of Virginia, 1998.

Halifax, Joan (ed.). *Shamanic Voices: A Survey of Visionary Narratives*. New York: Arkana, 1991.

Haraway, Donna. *When Species Meet*. Minneapolis, MN: University of Minnesota Press, 2008.

Hartmann, Heinz. *Ego Psychology and the Problem of Adaptation*. Translated by David Rapaport. New York: International Universities Press, 1977.

Huizinga, Johan. *Homo Ludens: A Study of the Play Element in Culture*. Boston, MA: Beacon Press, 1955.

Jaynes, Julian. *The Origin of Consciousness in the Breakdown of the Bicameral Mind*. Boston, MA: Houghton Mifflin Company, 1982.

Kendall, Stuart. "Introduction: Sediment of the Possible." In *The Cradle of Humanity: Prehistoric Art and Culture*, 9–32. Edited by Stuart Kendall. New York: Zone Books, 2009.

Kohut, Heinz. *How Does Analysis Cure?* Edited by Arnold Goldberg. Chicago, IL: The University of Chicago Press, 1984.

Kohut, Heinz. *The Restoration of the Self*. New York: International Universities Press, 1986.

Kristeva, Julia. *New Maladies of the Soul*. Translated by Ross Guberman. New York: Columbia University Press, 1995.

Laplanche, Jean. *Freud and the Sexual*. Edited by John Fletcher. Translated by John Fletcher, Jonathan House, and Nicholas Ray. New York: International Psychoanalytic Books, 2011.

Laplanche, Jean and J.-B. Pontalis. *The Language of Psychoanalysis*. Translated by Donald Nicholson-Smith. New York: W. W. Norton & Company, 1973.

Leroi-Gourhan, Andre. *Treasures of Prehistoric Art*. Translated by Norbert Guterman. New York: Harry N. Abrams Publishers, 1967.

Leroi-Gourhan, Andre. *Gesture and Speech*. Translated by Anna Bostock Berger. Cambridge, MA: MIT Press, 1993.

Levenson, Edgar A. *The Fallacy of Understanding: An Inquiry into the Changing Structure of Psychoanalysis*. New York: Basic Books, 1972.

Lévi-Strauss, Claude. "The Effectiveness of Symbols." In *Structural Anthropology*, 186–205. Edited and translated by Claire Jacobson. New York: Basic Books, 1963.

Lévi-Strauss, Claude. *The Elementary Structures of Kinship*. Translated by James H. Bell, John R. von Sturmer, and Rodney Needham. Boston, MA: Beacon Books, 1969/1949.

Lewin, Bertram D. "Sleep, the Mouth, and the Dream Screen." In *The Selected Writings of Bertram D. Lewin*, 87–100. Edited by Jacob A. Arlow. New York: Psychoanalytic Quarterly Press, 1973/1946.

Lewin, Bertram D. and Helen Ross. "Psychoanalytic Education: Syncretism." In *The Selected Writings of Bertram D. Lewin*, 484–491. Edited by Jacob A. Arlow. New York: Psychoanalytic Quarterly Press, 1973/1960.

Lewis-Williams, David. "Ethnographic Evidence Relating to 'Trance' and 'Shamans' among Northern and Southern Bushmen." In *South African Archaeological Bulletin*, 56–60. Vol. 47, 1992.

Lewis-Williams, David. *The Mind in the Cave: Consciousness and the Origins of Art.* London: Thames and Hudson, 2002.

Lingis, Alphonso. *Excesses: Eros and Culture.* Albany, NY: State University of New York Press, 1983.

Masson, Jeffrey M. *The Assault on Truth: Freud's Suppression of the Seduction Theory.* New York: Farrar, Straus and Giroux, 1984.

Nunberg, Herman. *Practice and Theory of Psychoanalysis, Volume II.* New York: International Universities Press, 1965.

Ott, Jonathan. *Pharmacotheon: Entheogenic Drugs, Their Plant Sources and History, 2nd Edition.* Kennewick, WA: Natural Products Co., 1996.

Pawlett, William. *Georges Bataille: The Sacred and Society.* New York: Routledge, 2016.

Racker, Heinz. *Transference and Counter-Transference.* Madison, CT: International Universities Press, 1991.

Ricciardi, Mirella. *Vanishing Africa.* London: Collins, 1974.

Richman, Michele. "Bataille's Prehistoric Turn: The Case for Heterology." In *Theory, Culture & Society*, 155–173. Vol. 35 (4–5), 2018.

Scarry, Elaine. *The Body in Pain: The Making and Unmaking of the World.* New York: Oxford University Press, 1985.

Schilder, Paul. *The Image and Appearance of the Human Body: Studies in the Constructive Energies of the Psyche.* New York: International Universities Press, 1978.

Spence, Donald. *Narrative Truth and Historical Truth: Meaning and Interpretation in Psychoanalysis.* New York: W. W. Norton & Company, 1982.

Spooner, Brian. "The Evil Eye in the Middle East." In *The Evil Eye*, 76–84. Edited by Clarence Maloney. New York: Columbia University Press, 1976.

Taussig, Michael. *Shamanism, Colonialism, and the Wild Man: Studies in Terror and Healing.* Chicago, IL: The University of Chicago Press, 1991.

Taussig, Michael. *The Nervous System.* New York: Routledge, 1992.

Taussig, Michael and Peter Lamborn Wilson. *Shamanism and Ayahuasca. Exit 18 Pamphlet Series.* Brooklyn, NY: Autonomedia, 2002.

Taylor, Mark. *Hiding.* Chicago, IL: The University of Chicago Press, 1997.

Tedlock, Dennis and Barbara Tedlock (eds). *Teachings from the American Earth: Indian Religion and Philosophy.* New York: Liveright Press, 1975.

Ungar, Steven. "Phantom Lascaux: Origin of the Work of Art." In *On Bataille*, 246–262. Edited by Allan Stoekl. *Yale French Studies.* Vol. 78, 1990.

Walsh, Roger and Charles S. Grob (eds). *Higher Wisdom: Eminent Elders Explore the Continuing Impact of Psychedelics.* Albany, NY: State University of New York Press, 2005.

Weiss, Allen S. *Perverse Desire and the Ambiguous Icon.* Albany, NY: State University of New York Press, 1994.

Williams, William Carlos. "Spring and All." In *The Red Wheelbarrow and Other Poems*, 3–8. Edited by William Carlos Williams. New York: New Directions, 2018/1923.

Wolinsky, Stephen. *Trances People Live: Healing Approaches in Quantum Psychology.* Falls Village, CT: The Bramble Company, 1991.

Young, James E. *The Texture of Memory: Holocaust Memorials and Meaning.* New Haven, CT: Yale University Press, 1993.

Part II

Psychotherapy with couples

Chapter 7

Sexual disgust redux

In a recent issue of *Psychoanalytic Dialogues*, Lawrence Josephs (2016) addressed the subject of sexual disgust in a paper titled "The Treatment of Oedipal Disgust: When One Person's Sexual Delight is Another's Disgust." Were it not for Josephs's claim to a "relational perspective" regarding the subject of sexual disgust along with its publication in *Psychoanalytic Dialogues: The International Journal of Relational Perspectives*, his treatment of sexual disgust might have slipped innocuously past my radar. However, on closer examination, the form and content of this article belies any notion of 'relational perspective' that I can conjure. Therefore, I offer a critical evaluation of Josephs's claim in the service of proposing an alternative understanding of what is meant by the term "relational" for clinicians. My response, accordingly, will be four-fold: I will first address the construction of Josephs discussion, particularly with regard to the use of references by which he authorizes his work. Second, contra Josephs's essay, I will propose an alternative understanding of a relational investigation. Third, I will apply this alternative relational perspective to a consideration of disgust, especially sexual disgust. Finally, through the lens of this alternative understanding, I consider Josephs's clinical material.

I. Critical evaluation of Josephs's argument

The explicitly stated impetus for Josephs's (2016) article is his contention that "sexual disgust has not been the object of much systematic theorizing within contemporary psychoanalysis despite the central role Freud assigned to disgust in the genesis of sexual repression" (411). Josephs goes on to suggest that "its undertheorization within the psychoanalytic literature" may be attributable to the sequence by which "the slightest possibility of exposure to a disgusting substance motivates reflexive physical as well as psychological avoidance" (418). His a priori speculations of this type are found throughout the article. To wit,

> Infidelity evokes moral disgust because it is perceived as a form of emotional abuse that humiliates the betrayed partner.

415

Unconsciously beauty is equated with goodness while ugliness is equated with badness.

417

Infidelity *may evoke* disgust because it constitutes coerced rather than voluntary partner sharing.

415 (emphasis added)

a relational theory of romantic desirability *suggests that* in a successful long-term relationship we can all potentially end up with a partner of uniquely high personal value to us that is superior to all others.

417 (emphasis added)

Some individuals are thought to be inherently disgusting because they are objectively ugly.

418

behavior that arouses sexual jealousy *may also* evoke disgust to shame the partner for seemingly unfaithful behavior that threatens attachment security.

419 (emphasis added)

Josephs's pervasive use of qualifiers notwithstanding (there are no fewer than 100 of such equivocating pre-modifiers, as emphasized in the preceding list, throughout his article), my position is that all the above statements are flatly culture-bound and ethnocentric. For Josephs's assertions to have relevance even within the confines of his own discipline and culture, to say nothing of cross-cultural validity, they must be inductively grounded in some form of empirical data. Instead, Josephs resorts to deductive speculation, primarily from three sources of authority: Freud's own scant writings directly addressing the subject of disgust; social psychology and cross-cultural psychology; and evolutionary psychology (other cognate psychoanalytic and popular psychology sources appear throughout). Because they serve as the basis of Josephs's arguments, I first examine some of these sources in detail:

The !Kung San

Josephs proposes that disgust is linked with sexual betrayal. He proceeds from his own prior work linking the primal scene to learned sexual behavior in other cultures (Josephs 2011, 2015). He states, "In fact, there are many cultures in which children learn about sex by watching their parents have sex (i.e. the primal scene) from a young age ... this is the way contemporary hunter-gatherer children still learn about sex" (2016, 415). The basis of this sweeping generalization is a single reference to anthropologist Melvin Konner's (2005) review of the literature on the !Kung San people of

Botswana. At no point in Konner's review article does he assert or support this statement. Moreover, Konner's comments express a very different sentiment than that implied by Josephs. Konner states, "Adults did not approve of sexual play [of children] and when it became obvious they discouraged it, usually by verbal chastisement ..." (30).

The !Kung San happen to be exceptionally well-studied by anthropologists and the ethnographic record regarding even this one group, let alone all hunting-gathering groups, simply does not support Josephs's assertion regarding the transmission of sexual knowledge via the primal scene. Ethnographer Lee (1979, 84), an authority on the !Kung San, observed, "parental sex is carried on discreetly while the children sleep"; ethnographer Shostak (1983, 105) commenting on the !Kung San states,

> Adults try to keep children from noticing their sexual activity, but arranging meetings in the bush is difficult and young children often insist on accompanying their mothers wherever they go. The alternative is to wait until the children are asleep, and try to be discreet;

and anthropologist Draper (1975, 83) adds, "The !Kung themselves claim that lovers (as well as married couples) sometimes arrange to meet privately in the bush. !Kung sleeping arrangements may promote these tactics, for at night whole families sleep outdoors together gathered around individual campfires."

Most importantly, few anthropologists or psychologists today easily agree that universal sexual behavior (or "disgusting" behavior for that matter) may be plausibly generalized on the basis of one society. Josephs's selection of ideal types that enable "scientific" deduction remains highly questionable as long as they are not inductively grounded in data that is both empirical and comparative. This may be additionally said of his reliance on such notions as "the environment of evolutionary adaptedness"; "the face" as a universal locus of signification; and his notion of "embodied moral cognition," all of which connote *reification*, a process with wide resonance that subsumes and ultimately contradicts Josephs's claim to a relational perspective.

The environment of evolutionary adaptedness (EEA)

Asserting how sexual knowledge is transmitted in "many cultures," Josephs (2016) states that children "emulate parental sexual relations through sexual play in the bushes with peers. This appears to be how children learned about sex in what Bowlby called 'the environment of evolutionary adaptedness,'" (415). Josephs valorizes his erroneous suppositions regarding sexual transmission by invoking a provisional if not outdated concept from Bowlby, namely, "the environment of evolutionary adaptedness" (hereafter, the EEA). Bowlby (1982, 59, emphasis added) states, the only relevant criterion by which to consider the natural adaptiveness of any particular part of present-day man's behavioral equipment is the degree to which and the way in which *it might* contribute to population survival in man's primeval environment.

These broad generalizations do not pass the test of scientific validity in light of current contributions from anthropology. Irons (1998, 196) states,

> In short, the EEA concept as currently used by evolutionary psychologists is unrealistic in terms of what is now known about human phylogeny, the pace of evolution, and the role of stabilizing selection in maintaining adaptations ... The difficulties with the EEA concept have to do primarily with paleontology and field observations of evolutionary change, subjects that [evolutionary psychologists] do not at all study in their empirical research.

Josephs's assertion implying the universal transmission of sexual knowledge by hunter-gatherers within the EEA neglects variance in space and time, across cultures and historical epochs, thereby conflating and essentializing human behavior for the purpose of making theoretical generalizations. His assertions are thus scientifically unreliable. Foley (1995, 195) remarks,

> Given the significance of variation for the operation of natural selection, it is important that [!Kung San] hunter-gatherer variability, both within and between groups, be used to elucidate adaptation rather than lost within a typological schema that seeks to characterize 'hunter-gatherer' as a uniform adaptation with uniform problems ... hunter-gatherers are themselves extremely variable in their ways of living. The so-called adaptive traits of hunter-gatherers should be treated as axes of variation rather than type.

The human face

Josephs (2016) suggests an inherent, genetic basis for specific expressions of the human face that he treats as universal markers of disgust: "Interestingly, the facial expression for disgust (i.e. crinkled upturned nose, open mouth, retracted upper lip, protruding lower lip, possibly extended tongue) is present at birth and appears to be elicited by certain smells or tastes" (411). He adds, "What appears to be preprogrammed are the facial expression for disgust ..." (412).

While Schilder (1978, 238–239) rightfully asserts the preeminence of the human face as "the most expressive part of the human body" ("the human face alone is capable of making some 250,000 different expressions" (Birdwhistle 1970, 9)), anthropologists devoted to the study of non-verbal behavior have concluded that "even before the development of kinesics, it became clear that this search for universals was culture-bound ... there are probably no universal symbols of emotional state" (Birdwhistle 1963, 126). Numerous recent studies from psychologists now concur, producing research that repudiates the notion of the human face as a marker of universally expressed emotions in favor of a culturalist perspective. To wit,

> In sum, our data directly show, for the first time, differences in the expectations of facial expression signals across diverse cultures, challenging notions of a universal language of emotion and revealing a source of potential confusion during cross-cultural communication.
>
> Jack, Caldara, and Schyns (2011, 25)

> Our findings indicate that perceptions of emotion are not universal, but depend on cultural and conceptual contexts.
>
> Gendron, van der Vyver, Roberson, and Barrett (2014, 251)

> These findings challenge the universality hypothesis that a face speaks for itself, lending support to a more 'constructed' perspective of emotional perception — one that's highly dependent on context cues (e.g. vocalizations, body language, or emotion words).
>
> Merluzzi (2014, 1)

The American Psychological Association itself has officially acknowledged the cultural relativity of facial affect expression: "... people from different cultures perceive happy, sad or angry facial expressions in unique ways, according to new research published by the American Psychological Association" (APA 2011, 1). In so doing, the discipline arrives at a point long accepted by most social scientists (see Goffman 1967; De Vos 1976; Geurts 2003).

There is much at stake in Josephs's supposition of universal facial meaning along with the generalized aesthetic attributions of beauty and ugliness that he asserts. In the absence of a widely accepted relativistic perspective, Josephs's reliance on "universal" aesthetic qualities of facial expression and interpretation amount to a reversion to physiognomy (see Browne 1985; Burrows and Schumacher 1990; Gamwell and Tomes 1995; Gilman 1996, who all comment on the physiognomic axiom "there must be a certain native analogy between the external varieties of the countenance and form, and the internal varieties of the mind" (Lavater 1866, 3). Following from the physiognomic correspondence between external expression and internal experience, Josephs arrives deductively at the heuristic notion of "embodied moral cognition" to explain the outer manifestations of disgust.

Embodied moral cognition

Josephs (2016) quotes research which *"suggested* that disgust *may* reflect embodied moral judgement" and accordingly concludes that "disgust embodies moral relationships" (412, emphasis added); that "since moral transgressions elicit disgust, moral cognition is designed by evolution to draw upon a primitive rejection response" (413); that there is a "tendency of sexual disgust to be experienced concretely as embodied cognition" (418); that "physical disgust, sexual disgust, aesthetic disgust, and moral disgust all *appear to be* unconsciously linked as forms of embodied cognition" (417, emphasis added); and finally, that "sexual disgust *may be* an adaptive form of embodied moral cognition" (416, emphasis added).

Nowhere is it clearer than in these statements that Josephs, by way of vulgar evolutionary speculation, is seeking to embody an emotional experience that he can then claim is universal. Coming from a psychoanalyst, as Josephs apparently is, one might wonder why the concept of a superego, critical introject, or persecuting self-representation, along with its internalization, needs to be embodied at all. It is exactly that seduction to embody psychological experience that preoccupied Freud with his Project (1966), which he ultimately abandoned, dismissing it as "a kind of madness" (Masson 1995, 152; Lothane 1998, 49). However, Josephs's effort to materially establish moral cognition, deny variance and variability among the !Kung San hunting-gathering people in favor of a single ideal type, and postulate a single face for a universal human expression of disgust are not merely forms of madness, they are all hallmarks of *reification*. It is to reification as the antithesis of relational processes that I now turn.

II. Reification versus relational process

Reification as production

Partridge (1959) traces the etymology of the verb "to reify" as derivative from "real," thus at root, meaning "to invest with reality, whence *reification*, is literally 'to make property of'"" (553, author's emphasis). For the purposes of the current discussion, I wish to focus on this dynamic, productive aspect of reification. The antinomy between reification as production process and relational processes is most famously addressed by Marx in *Capital* (1990), in which he focuses on the material commodity as representing a dual process: it both personifies the result of production while simultaneously obscuring the actual social relations of production behind its formation. Thus, reification occurs when "a relation between people takes on the character of a thing and thus acquires a "phantom-objectivity," an autonomy that seems so strictly rational and all-embracing as to conceal every trace of its fundamental nature: the relation between people" (Lukacs 1990, 83).

Ollman (1990) explains the ramifications of reification for social relations: "the relations between men are not only reified in their products; but these reified products interact with men so as to make what appeared false true" (200).

> What is revealed here is the denial of authorship, the denial of relationship, and the denial of the reciprocity of process to the point where the manifold armory of assumptions, leaps of faith and a priori categories are ratified as real and natural
>
> Taussig (1992, 88)

thus resulting in "the thingification of the world, persons, and experience" (84).

The "mystification" behind reification further implies the subtle, successful transformation of relationship into fetish. Geras (1971) states, "The mechanism of mystification consists in the collapsing of social facts into natural ones. In this way, the value form is fetishized" (6).

The fetish

The process of reification is made manifest for anthropologists and psychoanalysts alike in the form of the fetish. For both, it is the instrumental object par excellence constructed against death, loss, and/or the dissolution of the individual/group. It disavows loss in the displaced form of a material surrogate, a maneuver blatantly presented in Josephs's case material.

> The word Fetish is of Portuguese origin. Some derive it from 'feitico', i.e. something which is made by the hand, and is therefore regarded as artificial, and unnatural, and later the word comes to mean magical; others derive it from 'faticeira', i.e. 'witch', or from 'faticeiria', i.e. 'witchcraft'.
>
> Budge (1992, 15–16)

Tylor (1874, II, 144–145) notes the likeness between animism – "the doctrine of spirits in general" that he believed originated as a primitive response to death and loss – and the subordinate category of fetishism, "the doctrine of spirits embodied in, or attached to, or conveying influence through, certain material objects." Thus,

> a fetish is redolent with life. The idol is filled with a spirit; it speaks in the oracle. So the fetish, whether a medicine bag, or image, or claw of beast or bird, is filled with a spirit. This imaginary animation gives fetishism its power over the savage mind.
>
> Dorman (1881, 141–142)

Psychoanalytically speaking, Freud (1961) commented on how a fetish is "doubly derived from contrary ideas," that is, disavowal and displacement (157). (This double action of the fetish is also associated with transitional objects by Winnicott, 1974). It always entails both the disavowal of absence, whether that be the missing penis of mother or simply, the missing mother, and the substitution of a surrogate.

> The fetish always represents the penis, it is always a substitute for it, whether metaphorically (= it masks its absence) or metonymically (= it is contiguous with its empty place) ... the fetish signifies the penis as absent, it is its negative signifier; supplementing it, it puts a 'fullness' in place of a lack.
>
> Metz (1982, 71)

With regard to our present concern, "the fetish not only has a disavowal value, but also *knowledge value*" (Metz 1982, 76, author's emphasis); it ushers in "a fundamental province of human reality, the realm of the imaginary" (Lacan 1956, 267) and hence acquires sign value. Baudrillard (1981, 93) states that "fetishism is actually attached to a sign object, the object eviscerated of its substance and history." This evisceration of history and relation in the service of creation is the double action that most writers commenting on fetishism agree on.

According to Freud,

> The situation only becomes pathological when the longing for the fetish passes beyond the point of being merely a necessary condition attached to the sexual object and actually takes the place of the normal aim, and, further, when the fetish becomes detached from a particular individual and becomes the sole sexual object.
>
> (1957, 153–154)

Such an attachment potentially implies a belief in the authenticity of the world of displaced objects we inhabit, all the while forgetting the underlying relational whole that belies their authenticity.

> What then is truth? A movable host of metaphors, metonymics, and anthropomorphisms: in short, a sum of human relations which have been poetically and rhetorically intensified, transferred, and embellished, and which, after long usage, seems to a people to be fixed, canonical, and binding. Truths are illusions that we have forgotten are illusions; they are metaphors that have become worn out and have been drained of sensuous force, coins which have lost their embossing and are now considered as metal and no longer as coins.
>
> Nietzsche (1995, 84)

Finally, we encounter "the phenomenon that increasingly abstract ideas hold sway, i.e. ideas which increasingly take on the form of universality" (Marx and Engels 1988, 65).

In both the form and content of Josephs's essay, and particularly his case material, we witness the mystification resulting from the introduction of deduced ideas that are themselves fetishized and combined to "explain" disgust. However, an alternate way to comprehend the experience of disgust allows us to take into account the relational processes masked by the fetish products of Josephs's narrative.

Relational process

A relational perspective includes but is not limited to fetishized objects, nor constrained by reified internal or external human qualities in order to comprehend its subject. It considers the idea *as well as* the social relations behind its production. Greenberg and Mitchell (1983) state, "Although they are not compelled to by the premises of their model, relational/structure theorists do tend to *deemphasize constitutional factors*" (229, emphasis added). Moreover, Mitchell (1988, 17) states, "Mind has been redefined from a set of predetermined structures emerging from inside an individual organism to transactional patterns and internal structures derived from an interactive, interpersonal field." In the same vein Schafer (1976, 3) states, "It is high time we stopped using this mixed physiochemical and evolutionary biological language altogether ... more than omission, we require new elements and a new ordering of them ... up to the present time we have lacked an alternative."

This alternative direction is outlined by Aron (1996, 10–11): "relational theory is linked philosophically to the position that man is a social animal and that human satisfactions are realizable only within a social community"; "relational theory is essentially a contemporary eclectic theory anchored in the idea that it is the relationships (internal and external, real and imagined) that are central" (18). For the present discussion, "relationships" refer as much to the intellectual community involved in the production of knowledge as it does the clinical dyad. As such, a relational perspective not only serves a therapeutic goal but a critical one, for it can dissolve the disciplinary boundaries and conceptual structures that obscure underlying relational processes.

Building on Aron's outline, this author urges a further progression for a "relational" perspective, that is, a relational perspective not just negatively framed as a remedial reaction to the outdated limits of an authoritarian, one-person, one-directional drive psychology (see Mitchell 1988; Aron 1996; or Dupont 1995). A true relational perspective for psychoanalysis overcomes its parochial historical disciplinary limitations once it holistically incorporates the contributions of the cognate fields in the humanities, physical, and social sciences (see Freeman 1970, 53–54). Mauss (1979, 101) states, "It is the triple viewpoint [physiological, sociological, and psychological], that of the 'total man,' that is needed."

Thus a relational perspective regards qualities like disgust as a *total social phenomenon*: "social phenomena are not discrete; each phenomenon contains all the threads of which the social fabric is composed. In these *total* social phenomena all kinds of institutions find simultaneous expression: religious, legal, moral, and economic" (Mauss 1967, 1, author's emphasis). Thus, I am proposing that an actual *relational* approach to a phenomenon such as disgust be predicated on a holistic perspective that includes both its psychological and social manifestations. This requires, as Durkheim (1982) famously expressed, that we "give up making psychology in some way the focal point of [our] operations, the point of departure to which [we] must always return after [our] adventurous incursions into the social world" (135). Accordingly, disgust is here regarded relationally as a *social fact* and "the determining cause of a social fact must be sought among antecedent social facts and not [exclusively] among the states of individual consciousness" (134). For "each single relationship or fact is an appearance whose full meaning or reality is only articulated by integrating it theoretically within the total social structure" (Geras 1971, 10).

III. An alternate relational view of disgust

The term *disgust* derives etymologically from its Latin root *gustus* and later develops into *gust* (or gusto) – to taste or to relish (Partridge 1959, 271). The Latin *dis* translates as "apart" hence the European term disgust to indicate "apart from relish or taste" or "a taste apart." Therefore, disgust represents a category of objects, persons, actions, or experiences that have been set apart and, by virtue of its Other status, are deemed "loathsome or offensive" (Onions 1965, 526).

This "taste apart" was the obsessive focus of French social theorist Georges Bataille who characterized it as "the accursed share." By way of an introduction, Bataille's life and work certainly qualify him as a theoretician of disgust. Rejected from the early twentieth-century surrealist circle by Breton (1994) who characterized him as "an excremental philosopher," Bataille authored sophisticated pornographic novels that would presage his later theoretical writings (see Sontag 1983). Over a period of 30 years beginning around the end of the First World War, he published extensively, established prominent scholarly journals (*Documents* and *Critique*), and initiated highly influential intellectual study groups (*College of Sociology* and *Acephale*). Bataille has been widely acknowledged as a formative intellectual influence by Barthes, Lacan, Kristeva, Foucault, and Derrida; and with the translation of his work into English in the late twentieth century, he has been received in the United States with "immense urgency" (Nehamas 1989, 31).

Of particular note in the current context, Bataille is widely hailed as the unofficial father of post-structuralist thought whose corpus critically confronted the very process of reification described above. I contend that Bataille's writings, both in form and content, exemplify a model for a relational perspective on disgust, a perspective that Bataille defined as "heterological" (Bataille 1991a). He supported his work by reference to a wide range of sources including Marx, Nietzsche, Hegel, Sade, and Freud, as well as numerous anthropological, historical, religious, and literary texts. From this multidisciplinary perspective, writing against the parochial and privileged perspective of any single subject or discipline, Bataille considered those realms of human activity that transpire beyond the immediate, concrete, functional, and utilitarian needs attached to sexual and social reproduction, as by-products of the "restricted economy" of capitalism. Looking past the functionalism of Freud's Eros instinct or Darwin's survival of the most adaptively fit, Bataille focused particularly on human behavior that cannot be rationalized as serving useful, adaptive, or functional aims, but rather those activities considered excessive within a pre-modern "general economy." In so doing he laid the groundwork for the hypothetical equation between excess and disgust and proposed what Levi (1922, 35) grasped intuitively – that "excess produces disgust."

To be sure, this is not the first such effort to place disgust in a relational context. Angyal (1941) began his research with the assertion that "[disgust] cannot be adequately understood without considering the periphery, that is, the transition to and connection with related phenomena" (393). However, given Bataille's focus on disgust, his open engagement of diverse and varied sources to understand the phenomenon, and his assignment of disgust to a preeminent place in human life, I am privileging his perspective as a framework for depicting an alternate, relational understanding of disgust.

Regarding the centrality of disgust for the human experience, Bataille states,

> Spontaneous physical revulsion keeps alive in some indirect fashion at least the consciousness that the terrifying face of death, its stinking putrefaction, are to be identified with the sickening primary condition of life. For primitive people the moment of greatest anguish is the phase of decomposition [and] the close connections between decomposition, the source of an abundant surge of life, and death ... The generative power of corruption is a naïve belief responding to the mingled horror and fascination aroused in us by decay ... decay summed up the world we sprang from and return to, and horror and shame were attached both to our birth and to our death ... death will proclaim my return to seething life. Hence I can anticipate and live in expectation of that multiple putrescence that anticipates it's sickening triumph in my person.
>
> 1986, 56–57

This line of reasoning led Bataille to proclaim, "I believe that nothing is more important for us than that we recognize that we are bound and sworn to that which horrifies us most, that which provokes our most intense disgust" (Bataille 1988, 114). Moreover, Bataille (1988, 106) goes so far as to attribute the generation of all human social arrangements to disgust: "Everything leads us to believe that early human beings were brought together by disgust and by common terror, by an insurmountable horror focused precisely on what originally was the central attraction of their union."

For Bataille, disgust exists always as one part of a dyad with attraction and completes a relationship attributable to "the parallels perceived by the human mind between putrefaction and the various aspects of sexual activity ... the feeling of revulsion which set us against both end up mingling" (1986, 61). Thus Bataille (1988, 106) claims that the nucleus of all societies is the object of a "fundamental repulsion ... the social nucleus is, in fact, taboo, that is to say, untouchable and unspeakable, from the outset it partakes of the nature of corpses, menstrual blood, and pariahs."

This primal attraction that is coterminous with disgust seeks the death of the individual subject and the dissolution of all socially constructed meaning (in a similar vein see Kristeva, 1982, on "the abject"). However, this sought-after loss or dissolution has no telos beyond itself. According to Bataille, it is only through the ecstatic and/or orgasmic act of expenditure that the death of the subject is achieved. Again, this expenditure is necessarily devoid of any instrumental, rational purpose to which it stands opposed. Its objects are absolutely, by definition, fully dissociated from reproductive, adaptive purposes; hence, they are set apart by humans as excessive and experienced as disgusting. They are the accursed share. They are the by-products of war, non-procreative eroticism, festival, and the ultimate social form of expenditure, sacrifice. In sum, Bataille viewed human existence as inherently split, divided between production/accumulation/function for survival, that which we share with all animals, and expenditure/excess/waste, that which accounts for specific social behavior that distinguishes humans from other animals.

According to Bataille, the exclusion/expulsion of this socially designated "accursed share" is deliberate, even required, and often manifests as a shocking violent discharge (as in the case of sacrifice). "From the very first, it appears that sacred things are constituted by an operation of loss" (Bataille 1991b, 119). Bataille states,

> The notion of the heterogeneous foreign body permits one to note the elementary subjective identity between types of excrement (sperm, menstrual blood, urine, fecal matter) and everything that can be seen as sacred, divine, or marvelous: a half-decomposed cadaver feeing through the night in a luminous shroud can be seen as characteristic of this unity.

94

The interplay of this unity between sacred and profane is addressed by Bataille in the world of eroticism (1986); erotic literature (1993); the lives of saints (1991c); and the criminally deviant (1991d), among others.

Bataille contended that the enlightened, practical person today regards this human impulse to expend, as well as the attraction to this impulse, with repulsion, as a surviving uncanny vestige of an earlier primitive experience. By limiting his discussion solely to the so-called pragmatic and adaptive function of disgust, Josephs's essay stands as an example of the human dilemma which Bataille bemoaned – the modern wholesale dismissal of our attraction to the repulsive notion of expenditure and the immediate, unmediated "sovereign" experience it potentially provides. Bataille states,

> Even when he does not spare himself and destroys himself while making allowance for nothing, the most lucid man will understand nothing, or imagine himself sick: he is incapable of a *utilitarian* justification for his actions, and it does not occur to him that a human society can have, just as he does, an *interest* in considerable losses, in catastrophes that, *while conforming to well-defined needs*, provoke tumultuous depressions, crises of dread, and, in the final analysis, a certain orgiastic state.
>
> 117 (1991b; author's emphasis)

Adopting Bataille's conceptual scheme for use in the clinic implies an acceptance of an inherently dual human constitution including both the tendency to produce and accumulate – *to the point of excess* – and the necessity of expenditure. Without the latter, the modern individual suffers a form of existential constipation with efforts toward expenditure erroneously construed as pathology (cutting, binging, purging, gambling, consuming, drinking, self-mutilation, trichotillomania, etc.). A progressive, relationally oriented treatment would entail the identification and interpretation of the vicissitudes between these two forces as they interact within our restricted socioeconomic context that privileges only one.

The enduring tension between the positivist, cumulative forces of production and the negative, destructive character of expenditure informed Bataille's adoption of the Hegelian dialectic (Hegel 1977; Kojeve 1991). The value of this methodological instrument, typically understood through the sequence of thesis/structure>antithesis/antistructure>synthesis, was that it could potentially reinstate the exceptional contribution of the negative, excessive, and disgusting as an aspect of antithesis leading to synthesis. However, unlike Hegel, Bataille (1990) emphasized the negative aspect of the dialectic process through which relational processes are generated: "[Man] bears within him *Negativity*, and the force, the violence of negativity cast him into the incessant movement of history, which changes him and which alone realizes the totality of the concrete real over time" (12, author's emphasis).

Aron (1996, 264) reinforces the compatibility of the dialectical perspective for a relational investigation: "relational psychoanalysis asserts that analytic objectivity is constituted dialectically, rooted in the intersubjective relationship." It is through the dialectical and, particularly the under-valued role of the negative in the dialectical, that we now turn to Josephs's case material featuring his psychotherapeutic treatment of a couple.

IV. A couple's treatment revisited

Josephs (2016) concludes his discussion of sexual disgust with a presentation of his treatment of a couple. Consistent with his preceding review of the literature he claims that the treatment demonstrates how

> the phobic avoidance of sexual disgust can better be addressed by appreciating the adaptive relational functions of sexual disgust as embodied moral cognition and its origins in oedipal psychodynamics that unconsciously link disgust to morally offensive aspects of sexual relationships, like sexual betrayal, that threaten attachment security.
>
> 423

Hence, his presentation is framed as an affirming application of his foregoing theoretical inferences regarding disgust.

Josephs states at the outset that the couple placed him in a "highly conflicted position" (418). By positioning himself front and center in his presentation, we suppose, relationally speaking, that Josephs experienced his own distress regarding disgust as he entered the process. Josephs's preliminary conflict concerned his quandary regarding clinical situations "when one partner's sexual delight is the other partner's sexual disgust ... when empathy for one partner is likely to be perceived by the other as shaming or as coercive pressure to engage in disgusting sexual behavior" (418). Josephs acknowledged that while sexual disgust was "not the presenting problem, it may be lurking underneath the surface as an exceptionally shame sensitive issue that undermines attachment security and self-regard" (419). We are basically introduced to disgust as a problem that a) "seems impossible to negotiate" (419); and b) once (inevitably?) present in the treatment will need to be managed. For Josephs, the presence of disgust apparently correlated with concerns about coercion of one or more parties (including both members of the couple and the therapist). *His* concerns led to his explicitly identified goals of alleviating shame, insuring that all participants are "sufficiently safe," and creating a "more egalitarian relationship."

Josephs's opening concerns betray a definite idea about disgust that he, operating deductively, from the top down (as in his earlier theorizing), will bring to bear on his patients as well as us readers. From the previously discussed perspective of Bataille's work, Josephs's perspective exhibits all the trademarks of a "restricted economy." At no point are we openly encouraged to explore the attractive and potentially arousing features of what is excessive, unsafe, hierarchical, even humiliating – all corollaries of disgust located in the province of a "general economy." From the restricted economic perspective, the therapist's job is to balance the books, tie up loose ends, and leave no unexplained *excessive* remainder. Underlying this singular predisposition that equates balance, commensuration, and mental health, lies, I contend, a fear of excess and, by extension, disgust. Yet in spite of Josephs's value-laden approach the patients will attempt to include him in their dalliance with their potential delight in disgust. Hence the vignette becomes an account of how well he can convert their subterranean curiosity into the currency of his own conventional value structure.

Once Josephs establishes his agenda at the outset of treatment, the clinical narrative follows a straightforward dialectic featuring Thesis (patient David) – Antithesis (patient Susan) – Synthesis (therapist Josephs). This dialectic unfolds thematically in stages. In the first stage we encounter the instrumental nature of the treatment itself. David participates and invests heavily in "intensive long-term psychoanalysis," he wants Susan to enter long-term treatment like himself; Susan participates "in a psychoanalytic psychotherapy with CBT elements," she does not want to invest in long-term psychoanalysis. Josephs makes much of this conflict in the service of establishing his authority within both the treatment and the clinical narrative. He states that the split between psychoanalysis and psychotherapy, as distinct treatment methodologies, "has had a detrimental effect on the field in inhibiting psychotherapy integration and undermining the analyst's professional sense of identity when not practicing clinical psychoanalysis more narrowly defined" (419). Hence Josephs unapologetically rationalizes his authority as the synthesizer in the treatment room, claiming that his "more directive and didactic interventions can free patients from interpersonal vicious circles in a way that only interpreting the meaning of a relational dynamic might not" (419).

Once he possesses the authority in the room, Josephs, as synthesizer, promotes reciprocal acceptance in the face of the couple's conflict as he understands it. He does this by explicitly introducing an extraneous, fetishized object, a reified symbol of authority – the "embodied moral cognition." He states, "Appreciating that sexual disgust may be a form of embodied moral cognition lends itself to an acceptance approach in which disgust is appreciated as a moral sentiment that has its reasons" (419). The introduction of this notion following his appeal for acceptance has the predictable result. The couple are described as now accepting Josephs's authority, his wish for their acceptance of each other (and himself), and his deductively construed "evolutionary" explanation of their anxious conflict as regards the treatment.

The dialectic unfolds: Susan is tall, attractive, and prosperous; David is short, "reasonably attractive," and financially challenged by his expensive psychoanalytic treatment. David won't expend, he accuses Susan of treating him like "a sperm bank"; Susan becomes defensive when criticized. David wants more empathy for his generalized feelings of injury and Susan feels he should stop ruminating and move on. The couple alternately vacillates between giving and withholding. The economics of their conflict, both implicitly and explicitly, directly relate to the philosophy guiding the treatment process. Will Josephs help them balance the books, so to speak, or alternatively, explore their wish (of each other) to spend more freely, without regard for commensuration? Josephs elects the former by framing the couples' competing positions as different but equal, as consisting of "different coping strategies." He rationalizes his admittedly "didactic" stance by reference to a second deductively derived reified/fetishized construction, that is, another concept extraneous to the treatment process – "perspectival realism" (421). As with all hierarchical propositions, Josephs again affirms his own authority in the treatment interaction by reference to a transcendent principle (Rappaport 1971), one that is evidently solipsistic in nature (Hare 2017).

Eventually Susan, representing the negative aspect of the treatment dialectic and seeming to operate out of utter frustration, moved the treatment project forward with her resounding "No" to both David and Josephs, stating that she "no longer wanted to even try because it was just too much work and effort." When this resulted in David backing off, Josephs took this as proof that "they had both internalized and begun to independently apply the acceptance perspective as an 'observational platform,'" (421) (yet another reified/fetishized and experience-distant device). However, the autonomous, excessive, and non-commensurate impact of Susan's "No" is evidenced in what reportedly follows as the treatment focus shifts to sex.

The dialectic advances further: David wants more sex, stating he feels that Susan withholds due to unanalyzed repression. Susan, eschewing the psychoanalytic route to her sexuality, resents being patronized and mischaracterized. Josephs reiterates his appeal for mutual acceptance, this time focusing on the couples' disparate (but, of course, equally valid) sexual styles. However, the sexual differences discussion touches on the issue of sexual disgust with David wondering if his sexuality disgusts Susan. Josephs, ignoring (suppressing?) David's implicit wish suggests that both parties might feel disgust in relation to their sexual life with his implicit directive being to replace disgust with empathy. Nevertheless, Susan, actually far from being repressed, moved the treatment forward again by saying No to the mischaracterization of her as a prude – she "protested that she was open to being more sexually accommodating and experimental if David were to talk more openly about what he wanted" (422). Moreover, Susan further develops the sexual focus with a discussion, the only specific discussion of sexuality in this case material, of her previous sexual partner and his interest in sadomasochism, pornography, and role-playing. She characterized herself with this previous partner as "sexually withholding in a way that was disgustingly 'anal'" (423). Rather than view these statements psychoanalytically as unconscious derivatives of sexual desire, as an opening (in the fullest meaning of that word) to the rich world of female sexuality, they are interpreted by Josephs as a prelude to a "reparative experience [that] allowed Susan to feel sufficiently safe" (423).

At this point, I surmise that Josephs, David, and we readers are being made safe from the possible engagement with the potentially "disgusting," unexplored world of this couple's erotic life, moreover, safe from the world of Bataillean eroticism where either David or Susan or both might declare, "I don't want your love unless you know I am repulsive, and love me even as you know it" (Bataille 1966, 33). Quite the contrary; following Josephs's "reparative" engagement with Susan we learn in short order that the treatment is concluding – the couple are suddenly married and Susan is pregnant. However, in the closing words of the case vignette Josephs informs us that the couple "both had been raised as observant Jews" (423). This late revelation is especially significant considering the abrupt transition from the mention of Susan's sexuality to her married-with-child status. By invoking this social fact, Josephs rationalized the underlying restricted economics of his treatment goals. That is, Judeo-Christian culture is based on foundational tenets derived from the Torah and known as the Shulchan Aruch or, The Jewish Code of Law. Key among these tenets is Section Even Ha Ezer (23: 1) which states,

> It is prohibited to spill seed needlessly and this sin is more severe than all Torah transgressions. For this reason a man should not thresh inside and sprinkle [his semen] outside [of a woman], and he should not marry a girl who is unable to have children.

This sacred prohibition against non-procreative eroticism forecloses on any notion of erotic pleasure/expenditure without a productive goal for this couple. It prescribes productive procreation and proscribes eroticism.

Yet in spite of this religious rationalization for an exclusive commitment to (re)production, Susan asserts her non-productive wish to expend one last time. She insists on a bris for her male infant against the wishes of her husband. Reportedly, David fears the traumatic consequence of such a sacrifice. Josephs attributes this to David's disgust with the practice of ritual circumcision, though this disgust is not at all clear. I contend that as with his sperm earlier, David is withholding out of fear of expenditure and the loss it involves, a loss that he apparently associates with his wife's sexuality in the face of which he attests to feeling inadequate. However, Josephs (2016) redeems David in the final two sentences of the case that illuminate the actual purpose of this treatment: "Family lore had it that the mohel who had performed David's circumcision had messed it up. Yet Susan proudly testified that David's penis was perfectly normal looking, implicitly attempting to heal the narcissistic scar left by David's Oedipal self-disgust" (423).

Josephs ends the treatment with the couple finally in agreement over what apparently was at issue all along – the affirmation of a normal, aesthetically acceptable and functional penis in the face of David's castration anxiety. The content and form of Josephs's essay testify to the virtue of the reified, productive side of life, to the success of the fetish in banishing the experience of loss, castration, and non-productive eroticism, all as organized and depicted by Josephs in the penultimate climactic and resolving figure of David's "normal" penis. As in any morality tale, the figures of the sadomasochistic ex-boyfriend and the bumbling, butchering mohel were invoked as supporting, extruded Others who were only incidental, as is the infant, to the consecration of the penis and its sexually productive, morally correct role. Sexual disgust is thereby triumphantly accounted for and vanquished.

V. Conclusion

Josephs set out to address sexual disgust, a phenomenon that he felt is under-theorized in the psychoanalytic cannon, as well as the extant psychological literature, since Freud. This author agrees with Josephs on the central importance of sexual disgust though this object of inquiry ultimately eludes him. The problem is present in his initial aims. Although we are promised a relational inquiry Josephs is guided by a moral agenda. His quasi-religious task, in form and content, is hermeneutical and as such, "is construed as the restoration of meaning addressed to the interpreter in the form of a message. This type of hermeneutics is animated by faith" (Ricoeur 2016, xvii). Thus Freud's charter will be properly affirmed and reinstated, disgust will resume its proper position in the psychoanalytic canon, and the paradigm will again be restored (see Kuhn 1970, on the role of "specialists" who are devoted to the application of a visionary leader's revolutionary paradigm). Josephs's essay thus betrays the same dynamic of authority and devotion that isomorphically informed his treatment of the couple.

Yet ironically, by the very nature of his task, Josephs remains at odds with Freud whose own writing betrayed a very different hermeneutical task.

> [Freud's] hermeneutics is regarded as the demystification of meaning presented to the interpreter in the form of a disguise ... [it] is animated by suspicion, by a skepticism toward the given, and it is characterized by a distrust of the symbol as a dissimulation of the real ... [it] looks upon the contents of consciousness as in some sense false [and] aims to transcend this falsity through a reductive interpretation and technique.
>
> Ricoeur (2016, xvii)

To this end, Freud worked comparatively between clinical experience and a wide diversity of intellectual sources (see Timms 1988). Rather than restore the dominant paradigm, he disconcerted it through critical confrontation and a radical revision.

I have attempted to employ a "hermeneutics of suspicion" in my critique of Josephs's discussion which I have juxtaposed with the thought of Georges Bataille. To this end, my review is offered as a remedial response to the reifications of that psychoanalytic treatment and exposition that is grounded in commensurate and efficient productivity. The perspective promoted is a direct engagement with excess and disgust – with both one's patients, oneself, and one's society – and extends my previous focus on the generative power of the negative (Buse 2006). As Lichtenberg (2008) expresses it, "An analyst's reaction of disgust-revulsion or startle-revulsion when triggered by the particular sexual practices adopted by their patients in an effort to break free of problematic inhibitions challenges the analyst to examine his or her own Eew! Factor" (9–10).

Through the form of this essay I have also sought to express a relational basis for our knowledge; not just dialectically in the treatment room, but dialogically with a diverse range of disciplines; not just between Josephs and myself, but through ethnographic conversation with other cultures. To this end, I have invoked the specters of Marx, Nietzsche, and Freud, who each addressed the human tendency to invest our fetishized ideas with lives of their own. Josephs's non-critical, non-relational reliance on reified, culture-bound constructions are a case in point, demonstrating that "to make a premise 'self-evident' is the simplest way to make action based upon that premise seem 'natural'" (Bateson 1976, 63). I propose that an actual excursion into the anthropological literature, again, after the model of Freud (see Wallace 1983), might help us avoid such ethnocentrism and enhance our idea of what we mean when we speak about "relational" processes. In the meantime, to Josephs and his readers, I echo the sentiment of anthropologist Gregory Bateson, who warned, "What is disastrous is to claim an objectivity for which we are untrained and then project upon an external world premises that are either idiosyncratic or culturally limited" (Bateson 1976, 55).

Bibliography

American Psychological Association. "Perception of Facial Expressions Differs across Cultures." 2011. Press release. Retrieved from www.apa.org/print-this.aspx.

Angyal, Andras. "Disgust and Related Aversions." In *Journal of Abnormal and Social Psychology*, 393–412. Vol. 36 (3), 1941.

Aron, Lewis. *A Meeting of Minds: Mutuality in Psychoanalysis.* Hillsdale, NJ: Analytic Press, 1996.

Bataille, Georges. *Erotism: Death & Sensuality,* Translated by Mary Dalwood. San Francisco, CA: City Lights Books, 1986/1957.

Bataille, Georges. "Attraction and Repulsion II." In *The College of Sociology 1937–39*, 113–124. Edited by Denis Hollier. Translated by Betsy Wing. Minneapolis, MN: University of Minnesota Press, 1988/1938.

Bataille, Georges. "My Mother." In *My Mother/Madame Edwarda/The Dead Man*, 23–134. Translated by Austryn Wainhouse. New York: Marion Boyars, 1989/1966.

Bataille, Georges. "Hegel, Death, and Sacrifice." In *On Bataille*, 9–28. Edited by Allan Stoekl. Translated by Jonathan Strauss. New Haven, CT: Yale French Studies. Vol. 78, 1990/1955.

Bataille, Georges. "The Use Value of D. A. F. de Sade." In *Visions of Excess: Selected Writings, 1927–1939*, 91–104. Edited and translated by Allan Stoekl. Minneapolis, MN: University of Minnesota, 1991a/1930.

Bataille, Georges. "The Notion of Expenditure." In *Visions of Excess: Selected Writings, 1927–1939*, 116–129. Edited and translated by Allan Stoekl. Minneapolis, MN: University of Minnesota Press, 1991b/1933.

Bataille, Georges. *The Impossible*. Translated by Robert Hurley. San Francisco, CA: City Lights Books, 1991c/1962.

Bataille, Georges. *The Trial of Gilles de Rais*. Translated by Richard Robinson. Los Angeles, CA: AMOK Books, 1991d/1965.

Bataille, Georges. *Literature and Evil*. Translated by Alastair Hamilton. New York: Marion Boyars Publishers, 1993/1957.

Bateson, Gregory. "Some Components of Socialization for Trance." In *Socialization as Cultural Communication: Development of a Theme in the Work of Margaret Mead*, 51–63. Edited by Theodore Schwartz. Berkeley, CA: University of California Press, 1976.

Baudrillard, Jean. *For a Critique of the Political Economy of the Sign*. Translated by Charles Levin. Candor, NY: Telos Press, 1981.

Birdwhistle, Ray. "The Kinesic Level in the Investigation of the Emotions." In *Expression of the Emotions in Man*, 123–139. Edited by P. H. Knapp. New York: International Universities Press, 1963.

Birdwhistle, Ray. *Kinesics and Context: Essays on Body Motion Communication*. New York: Ballantine Books, 1970.

Bowlby, John. *Attachment and Loss, Volume 1, 2nd Edition*. New York: Basic Books, 1982.

Breton, Andre. "Second Manifesto of Surrealism." In *Manifestoes of Surrealism*, 117–194. Edited by Jean-Jacques Pauvert. Translated by Richard Seaver and Helen R. Lane. Ann Arbor, MI: University of Michigan Press, 1994/1930.

Browne, Janet. "Darwin and the Face of Madness." In *The Anatomy of Madness: Essays in the History of Psychiatry, Volume 1*, 151–165. Edited by W. F. Bynum, Roy Porter, and Michael Shepherd. New York: Tavistock Publications, 1985.

Budge, Sir E. A. Wallis. *Amulets and Talismans*. New York: Citadel Press, 1992/1968.

Burrows, Adrienne and Iwan Schumacher. "The Physiognomy of Insanity." In *Portraits of the Insane: The Case of Dr. Diamond*, 35–49. Edited by Adrienne Burrows and Iwan Schumacher. New York: Quartet Books, 1990.

Buse, William. "Toward a Genealogy of Psychoanalysis." In *Psychoanalytic Review*, 521–540. Vol. 93 (4), 2006.

De Vos, George A. "Affective Dissonance and Primary Socialization: Implications for a Theory of Incest Avoidance." In *Socialization as Cultural Communication: Development of a Theme in the Work of Margaret Mead*, 73–90. Edited by Theodore Schwartz. Berkeley, CA: University of California Press, 1976.

Dorman, Rushton. *The Origin of Primitive Superstitions and Their Development into the Worship of Spirits and the Doctrine of Spiritual Agency among the Aborigines of America*. London: J. R. Lippincott & Company, 1881.

Draper, Patricia. "Kung Women: Contrasts in Sexual Egalitarianism in Foraging and Sedentary Contexts." In *Toward an Anthropology of Women*, 77–109. Edited by Rayna R. Reiter. New York: Monthly Review Press, 1975.

Durkheim, Émile. *The Rules of Sociological Method*. Translated by W. D. Halls. New York: Free Press, 1982/1895.

Foley, Robert. "The Adaptive Legacy of Human Evolution: A Search for the Environment of Evolutionary Adaptedness." *Evolutionary Anthropology*, 194–203. Vol. 4 (6), 1995.

Freeman, Derek. "Totem and Taboo: A Reappraisal." In *Man and His Culture: Psychoanalytic Anthropology after "Totem and Taboo"*, 53–80. Edited by Werner Muensterberger. New York: Taplinger Publishing Company, 1970.

Freud, Sigmund. "Three Essays on the Theory of Sexuality." In *The Standard Edition of the Complete Psychological Works of Sigmund Freud, Volume VII*, 123–245. Edited and translated by James Strachey. London: Hogarth Press, 1957/1905.

Freud, Sigmund. "Fetishism." In *The Standard Edition of the Complete Psychological Works of Sigmund Freud, Volume XXI*, 147–157. Edited and translated by James Strachey. London: Hogarth Press, 1961/1927.

Freud, Sigmund. "Project for a Scientific Psychology." In *The Standard Edition of the Complete Psychological Works of Sigmund Freud, Volume I*, 283–387. Edited and translated by James Strachey. London: Hogarth Press, 1966/1895.

Gamwell, Lynn and Nancy Tomes. *Madness in America: Cultural and Medical Perceptions of Mental Illness before 1914*. Ithaca, NY: Cornell University Press, 1995.

Gendron, Maria, Jacoba M. van der Vyver, Debi Roberson, and Lisa F. Barrett. "Perceptions of Emotions from Facial Expressions Are Not Culturally Universal: Evidence from a Remote Culture." In *Emotion*, 251–262. Vol. 14 (2), 2014.

Geras, Norman. "Essence and Appearance: Aspects of Fetishism in Marx's 'Capital'." *New Left Review*, I/65, January–February 1971. Retrieved from https://newleftreview-org.ezproxy.cul.columbia.edu/I/65/norman-geras.

Geurts, Kathryn L. *Culture and the Senses: Bodily Ways of Knowing in an African Community*. Berkeley, CA: University of California Press, 2003.

Gilman, Sander L. *Seeing the Insane*. Lincoln, NE: University of Nebraska Press, 1996.

Goffman, Erving. "On Face-work." In *Interaction Ritual: Essays on Face-to-Face Behavior*, 5–45. Edited by Erving Goffman. Garden City, NY: Anchor Books, 1967.

Greenberg, Jay R. and Stephen A. Mitchell. *Object Relations in Psychoanalytic Theory*. Cambridge, MA: Harvard University Press, 1983.

Hare, Caspar. *On Myself, and Other Less Important Subjects*. Princeton, NJ: Princeton University Press, 2017.

Hegel, Georg W. F. *Phenomenology of Spirit*. Translated by A. V. Miller. New York: Oxford University Press, 1977/1807.

Irons, William. "Adaptively Relevant Environments versus the Environment of Evolutionary Adaptiveness." In *Evolutionary Anthropology*, 194–204. Vol. 6 (6), 1998.

Jack, Rachael E., Robert Caldera, and Philippe G. Schyns. "Internal Representations Reveal Cultural Diversity in Expectations of Facial Expressions of Emotion." In *Journal of Experimental Psychology*, 19–25. Vol. 141 (1), 2011.

Josephs, Lawrence. "The Primal Scene in Cross-species and Cross-cultural Perspectives." In *International Journal of Psychoanalysis*, 1263–1287. Vol. 92 (5), 2011.

Josephs, Lawrence. "How Children Learn about Sex: A Cross-species and Cross-cultural Analysis." *Archives of Sexual Behavior*, 1059–1069. Vol. 44 (4), 2015.

Josephs, Lawrence. "The Treatment of Oedipal Disgust: When One Person's Sexual Delight Is Another's Disgust." *Psychoanalytic Dialogues*, 410–426. Vol. 26 (4), 2016.

Kojeve, Alexandre. *Introduction to the Reading of Hegel: Lectures on the "Phenomenology of Spirit"*. Assembled by Raymond Queneau. Edited by Allan Bloom, Translated by James H. Nichols, Jr. Ithaca, NY: Cornell University Press, 1991/1947.

Konner, Melvin. "Hunter-Gatherer Infancy and Childhood: The !Kung and Others." In *Hunter-Gatherer Childhoods: Evolutionary, Developmental, and Cultural Perspectives*, 19–64. Edited by B.S. Hewlett and M. E. Lamb. New Brunswick, NJ: Aldine Transaction, 2005.

Kristeva, Julia. *Powers of Horror: An Essay on Abjection*. New York: Columbia University Press, 1982.

Kuhn, Thomas. *The Structure of Scientific Thinking, 2nd Edition*. Chicago, IL: The University of Chicago Press, 1970.

Lacan, Jacques. "Fetishism: The Symbolic, the Imaginary, and the Real." In *Perversions: Psychodynamics and Therapy*, 265–276. Edited by Sandor Lorand and Michael Balint. New York: Gramercy Publishing Company, 1956.

Lavater, Johann C. *Physiognomy: Or the Corresponding Analogy between the Confirmation of the Features and the Ruling Passions of the Mind*. London: William Tegg, 1866.

Lee, Richard B. *The Dobe !Kung*. New York: Holt, Rinehart and Winston, 1979.

Levi, Eliphas. *The Paradoxes of the Highest Sciences*. Chennai: Theosophical Publishing House, 1922.

Lichtenberg, Joseph D. *Sensuality and Sexuality across the Divide of Shame*. New York: Analytic Press, 2008.

Lothane, Zvi. "Freud's 1895 'Project': From Mind to Brain and Back Again." In *Annals of the New York Academy of Sciences*, 43–65. Vol. 843, 1998.

Lukacs, Georg. *History and Class Consciousness: Studies in Marxist Dialectics*. Cambridge, MA: MIT Press, 1990/1922.

Marx, Karl and Friedrich Engels. *The German Ideology*. Edited by C. J. Arthur. Translated by W. Lough. New York: International Publishers Co., 1988/1846.

Marx, Karl. *Capital: A Critique of Political Economy, Volume 1*. Translated by Ben Fowkes. New York: Penguin Books, 1990/1867.

Masson, Jeffrey M. (ed. and trans.). *The Complete Letters of Sigmund Freud to Wilhelm Fliess, 1887–1904*. Cambridge, MA: Belknap Press of Harvard University Press, 1995.

Mauss, Marcel. *The Gift: Forms and Functions of Exchange in Archaic Societies*. Translated by Ian Cunnison. New York: W. W. Norton & Company, 1967/1925.

Mauss, Marcel. "The Notion of Body Techniques." In *Sociology and Psychology: Essays by Marcel Mauss*, 95–105. Translated by Ben Brewster. Boston, MA: Routledge & Kegan Paul, 1979/1935.

Merluzzi, Andrew. "Nonverbal Accents: Cultural Nuances in Emotion Expression." In *Observer*, Vol. 27 (4) Association for Psychological Science, 2014. Retrieved from www.psychologicalscience.org/index.php/publications/observer/2014/april-14/nonverbal-accents.html.

Metz, Christian. *The Imaginary Signifier: Psychoanalysis and the Cinema*. Translated by Celia Britton, Annwyl Williams, Ben Brewster, and Alfred Guzzetti. Bloomington, IN: Indiana University Press, 1982.

Mitchell, Stephen. *Relational Concepts in Psychoanalysis: An Integration*. Cambridge, MA: Harvard University Press, 1988.

Nehamas, Alexander. "The Attraction of Repulsion: The Deep and Ugly Thought of Georges Bataille," In *The New Republic*, 31–36. October 23, 1989.

Nietzsche, Friedrich. "On the Truth and Lies in a Non-moral Sense." In *Philosophy and Truth: Selections from Nietzsche's Notebooks of the Early 1870's*, 79–97. Edited and translated by Daniel Breazeale. Atlantic Highlands, NJ: Humanities Press, 1995/1873.

Ollman, Bertell. *Alienation: Marx's Conception of Man in Capitalist Society, 2nd Edition*. Cambridge: Cambridge University Press, 1990.

Onions, Charles T. (ed.). *The Shorter Oxford English Dictionary of Historical Principles*. London: Oxford University Press, 1965.

Partridge, Eric. *Origins: A Short Etymological Dictionary of Modern English*. New York: Macmillan, 1959.

Rappaport, Roy. "The Sacred in Human Evolution." In *Annual Review of Ecology and Systematics*, 23–34. Vol. 2, 1971.

Ricoeur, Paul. *Hermeneutics and the Human Sciences*. New York: Cambridge University Press, 2016.

Schafer, Roy. *A New Language for Psychoanalysis*. New Haven, CT: Yale University Press, 1976.

Schilder, Paul. *The Image and Appearance of the Human Body: Studies in the Constructive Energies of the Psyche*. New York: International Universities Press, 1978.

Shostak, Marjorie. *Nisa: The Life and Words of a !Kung Woman*. New York: Vintage Books, 1983.

Shulchan Arukh, Even HaEzer 23:1. Retrieved from www.sefaria.org/Shulchan_Arukh,_Even_HaEzer.23?lang=bi.

Sontag, Susan. "The Pornographic Imagination." In *The Susan Sontag Reader*, 205–233. Edited by Raymond James Sontag. New York: Vintage Books, 1983.

Taussig, Michael. "Reification and the Consciousness of the Patient." In *The Nervous System*, 83–109. Edited by Michael Taussig. New York: Routledge, 1992.

Timms, Edward. "Freud's Library and His Private Reading." In *Freud in Exile: Psychoanalysis and Its Vicissitudes*, 65–79. Edited by Edward Timms and Naomi Segal. New Haven, CT: Yale University Press, 1988.

Tylor, Edward B. *Primitive Culture: Researches into the Development of Mythology, Philosophy, Religion, Language, Art, and Custom*. New York: Henry Holt and Company, 1874.

Wallace, Edwin R. *Freud and Anthropology: A History and Reappraisal*. New York: International Universities Press, 1983.

Winnicott, Donald W. *Playing and Reality*. New York: Penguin Books, 1974.

Part III

Psychotherapy with groups

Chapter 8

The acephalic stage

This chapter introduces the developmental notion of an acephalic stage. The acephalic stage exists as a potential in the process of any social group. It is realized through a transgressive act that ruptures the integrity of the group and, in so doing, distinguishes between a collection of individuals who communicate and those who have achieved community. The terms used here to frame the group process – acephale, transgression, community – reflect a deliberate effort to apply the theoretical ideas of social theorist Georges Bataille within the clinical setting and, by extension, to suggest the relevance of these ideas to social life in general.

The acephale is a French term that denotes that which is headless, usually with reference to a human body without a head. The image of the acephale is occasionally invoked as a symbol that suggests a reversal of the usual, familiar relationship, that is, the dominance of the executive head over the servility of the base or body. Insofar as the acephale has overcome the dominant values and privilege associated with the head, it represents freedom from a restrictive hierarchy.

This might be understood as social freedom in the case of the societies identified as "acephalic" by anthropologist E. Evans-Pritchard (1967). When he encountered an acephalic form of political system among the Nuer of Africa he thought he had found a relic of humankind's earliest form of government. "A Nuer tribe might be called acephalic in the sense they recognized a common rule of law but it would be hard to recognize any person with recognized responsibility for coordinating public activities throughout the tribe" (Mair 1972, 117).

Although Evans-Pritchard invoked the acephale to metaphorically represent our earliest form of social life, the acephale serves equally as a potent symbol for our future. A future, as imagined by Nietzsche (1968, 9), that is characterized by a necessary transitional stage of nihilism to come when "the highest values devaluate themselves."

Influenced by early anthropological accounts as well as Nietzsche, Marx, Hegel, and a wide array of other literary and scientific sources, Georges Bataille constructed his own theory of social life around the figure of the acephale. Best known as a social theorist, surrealist, and pornographer, Bataille first unearthed the symbol of the acephale in his study of medieval Gnosticism. There he sought to associate the base figure of the acephale with that which is sacred:

> Base matter is external and foreign to ideal human aspirations, and it refuses to allow itself to be reduced ... the psychological process brought to light by Gnosticism had the same impact: it was a question of disconcerting the human spirit and idealism before something base, to the extent that one recognized the helplessness of superior principles.
>
> 1991a, 51

Developing his focus on the subversive power of base matter, Bataille first set out to rewrite the body in articles entitled: The Solar Anus; The Big Toe; Rotten Sun; Mouth; and The Pineal Eye. Bataille's exploration eventually led to the coalescence of a secret society whose journal, entitled *Acephale*, published its own mission statement. Among its goals were to,

> Realize the universal accomplishment of personal being in the irony of the animal world and through the revelation of an acephalic universe, one of play, not of state or duty;
> Take upon oneself perversion and crime, not as exclusive values, but as integrated within the human totality;
> Fight for the decomposition and exclusion of all communities – nationalist, socialist, communist, or churchly – other than universal community ....
>
> 1986, 79

It was no random exercise that led Bataille to form the secret society, Acephale. Rather, the inspiration grew from Bataille's preoccupation with the restrictive aspects of contemporary social arrangements that offered a highly limited and culture-bound definition of what it means to be human. This led to his interest in anthropology and especially the secret society as a social form "to which recourse is always possible when the primary organization of society can no longer satisfy all the desires that arise" (Caillois 1988, 149). Bataille here is echoing a similar sentiment expressed earlier by Simmel (1950, 347) who suggested that

> the secret society emerges everywhere as the counterpart of despotism and police restriction, as the protection of both the defensive and offensive in their struggle against the overwhelming pressures of central powers – by no means of political powers only, but also of the church, as well as of school classes and families.

The image of the acephale bears an affinity to the notion of a secret society. They both express a social experience that resists and evades explanation by conventional sociological narratives (for the definitive presentation of the secret society of *Acephale* see Bataille 1995; Galletti and Brotchie 2017).

Conventional notions of society posit that groups exist functionally to optimize reproductive success against the threat of death. To this end, the leader fulfills an executive organizational function that includes administering, preserving, and representing the integrity and vitality of the group. In contrast, Bataille argued that this functionalist notion of society based on survival is specific to the scarcity and accumulation model of capitalism. He pointed to anthropological studies of the Aztecs and the Kwakiutl as illustrating other possible social arrangements that are organized instead around the notion of "expenditure" (see Bataille 1991b). By privileging this notion of expenditure, the group is then seen as an opportunity for each member to expend themselves and their individual identities, an action resulting in a visceral experience of loss through void, wound, or rupture that opens the possibility for what Bataille refers to as community. Again, contrary to conventional wisdom, this is not a vision of group as a defensive collection against death but rather as a vehicle through which death may be met and experienced – particularly if what is meant by death is the dissolution, the potentially orgiastic dissolution, of individual and private boundaries within and around the collective (varying explorations of Bataille's notion of community may be found in Blanchot 1988; Nancy 1991; Hegarty 2000; Mitchell and Winfree 2009).

According to Bataille, the expenditure par excellence for achieving community is sacrifice, particularly the sacrifice of the leader. This ultimate act enables the unmediated experience of community made possible when individual boundaries dissolve. Although Bataille references prehistoric societies, the modern ramifications for community may be glimpsed when a leader is sacrificed symbolically, as in the ritual celebration of crucifixion; metaphorically, as in Freud's (1957) imagined enactment of the primal Oedipal slaughter scenario; or literally, as in the case of the historical encounter between the French aristocracy and the guillotine. Above all, the sacrifice has to be non-productive and non-directed by functional aims that would tie it to a goal devised by and for a higher purpose. For if the sacrifice served a directed, functional aim, it would defeat the egalitarian prerequisite to the experience of community where, in the words of Canetti (1993, 15–16) "all are equal there, no distinctions count ... suddenly it is as though everything were happening in one and the same body."

The specific social techniques by which Bataille's notion of community is conjured consist of play, eroticism (sex without a reproductive purpose), festival, and sacrifice. In earlier human social arrangements, as noted by Durkheim (1995), community consisted of all these activities performed simultaneously on sacred occasions (resulting in what Durkheim famously refers to as "collective effervescence") – all characterized by their excessive nature in strong contrast with the rest of tribal life which was relatively profane, mundane, and based on efficient production. The opportunities for an experience of this type in modern times for any group are now limited, if not non-existent. Yet my experience as a clinician working within groups has presented me with an opportunity to explore the contemporary relevance of Bataille's vision of community based on expenditure.

In each group I have been a participant/observer in, there is a process that culminates in a moment during which the group members may elect to collectively terminate the authority of the group leader. This is an inevitable outcome of the realization that the leader cannot "satisfy all the desires that arise." Whether the leader is complicit or not, this excising of his or her authority reverberates through the group as an unmediated experience of its collective existence. This group sacrifice of its leader, along with its accompanying pattern of hierarchical governance, I refer to as the acephalic stage.

The ensuing post-leader experience belongs to the headless body, or what Bataille would associate with the base or big toe; what Nietzsche (1967) might speak of as the herd; or what Kristeva (1982) might refer to as the abject. There are many more potential outcomes to this process than I can possibly address here (I refer the reader to de Heusch (1982), Foucault (1977), and Girard (1977), to name but a few). What is of concern in the current context is whether or not the group experience of the acephalic stage holds the potential for an experience of community, that preeminent experience of the collective beyond the individual, as defined by Bataille. I should add that any effort to inculcate or foster this stage as a therapeutic goal (see Noys 2005) mitigates against the prerequisite possibility of an experience emerging from non-productive expenditure.

The following two case examples elucidate the acephalic stage and the group context from which it emerged. Both groups have a membership of psychotherapists as these are the groups most familiar to the author over the past 35 years. However, it is suggested here that the processes described are ubiquitous, transcend the experience of the two professionally defined groups discussed here, and have broad potential application depending on any group leader's ability to tolerate and equate success with their own marginalization within the group.

Case example I

The coalescence of a group of psychotherapists for the purpose of studying performers created the conditions conducive to the experience of the acephalic stage. The following is a brief chronology of their journey as it occurred in stages over 15 years:

1   *The psychotherapy service group*: The administration of the Postgraduate Center for Mental Health in New York City summoned a group of

psychotherapists from within their own community and set a mandate: establish a psychotherapy service entitled the Institute for Performing Artists (IPA) and determine through your clinical work if this population exhibits any extraordinary or special needs that justify the service you have established. The service provided individual and group psychotherapy to professional performers which served as the data from which their research proceeded. The group of therapists met once weekly to discuss their work and ideas for the duration of its 20-year existence. Its history included a changing composition of members and only two different leaders, one of which was the author.

2 *The search for an object*: The first group meeting of the IPA was characterized by collective dread for our existence as our survival depended on our ability to find an object that needed our services. To rationalize our endeavor we turned to the theoretical literature. Fenichel's paper (1946) "On acting" lent a Freudian affirmation. However, rejecting the focus on pathology typical of psychoanalytic studies like this we decided to emphasize the constructive or constitutive activity of acting. We did this by adopting the metaphor of the personal myth, that is, a characteristic, idiosyncratic enactment of an individual that is at once real and fantastic (see Decosta, Buse, and Amdursky 1986). While we still adhered to the Freudian view of these enactments as sublimations that were gratified through staged drama, we were suggesting that what was once considered a pathological construction was in fact a restitutive enactment. Having located an object, we (the IPA) could then describe it from a variety of psychoanalytic perspectives yet we never answered the vexing original question as to what, if any special attributes, set this population apart from all others. Did not all members of society possess and perform a personal myth? This stage lasted for ten years.

3 *The countertransference to the object*: Taking a different tack the IPA decided to explore the issues particular to performers through an exclusive focus on the type of countertransference inculcated in the therapist. It was hypothesized that this population, possibly more than others, exerted an unusually strong pull on the subject of the analyst to transgress the analytic frame required to conduct a psychoanalytically oriented treatment, for example, attend performances, observe monologues, read poems and scripts, and view tapes. When we each began sharing our incidents of transgression the group process ground to a halt which seemed to indicate a great deal of shame about revealing these extra-parameter events. This stage covered approximately four months.

4 *The transference to the object*: On exploring the inhibitions around the revelation of our transgressions we made an unexpected discovery. Everyone in our group had entertained some wish to be a performer themselves and most of the group had actualized these wishes through some type of performing activity. This could easily have curtailed the

process of our inquiry if we had settled for a Kohutian interpretation, that is, that we were inhibited due to a group resistance to revealing our own unacceptable exhibitionistic strivings (or for that matter, a Freudian interpretation in which our shame was reflective of our guilt at acting out our own wishes vis-à-vis the patient's seductive coercion). Instead we deferred any familiar and possibly reductionistic interpretation in favor of seeing what else might occur in the group. This stage of self-revelation regarding our own performing backgrounds lasted for one week.

5   *The search for the subject*: Abandoning our focus on the object all together we began focusing even more intently on the analyst's side of the equation. The group concluded that it could never really know the patients in any meaningful way outside of the analyst's case presentation and, by extension, the analyst himself or herself. Case presentations in our group meetings were rethought as performances thus casting other non-presenting group members into roles more like audience members, and gradually, as fellow performers. It was proposed that perhaps our patients were incidental to our meetings and that we were convening for the more fundamental purpose of constituting ourselves, or, as one of many such groups meeting within the Postgraduate Center, for the purpose of constituting our professional home. Patients were regularly brought in and sacrificed for this purpose, our purpose, our identity. The uncomfortable solipsistic possibilities suggested during this stage emerged intermittently for about four months.

6   *The objectification of the subject*: If everything that occurred in our group experience could be thought of as a type of aesthetic production or performance, where then was the authority to determine what is reality? This brought about a more far-reaching concern: suppose our reality is simply manufactured by drawing a frame around certain human activities and calling them performance/art. This art activity as staged, as framed, would then implicitly always be dialectically producing reality in so far as there existed an area outside the frame that is not-art. The despair attendant on this disorientation of our original a priori clinical assumptions was such that the group devoted itself to securing authorities in the form of professional experts from the world outside our space. The outstanding irony resulting from this was that noted author and psychoanalyst Adam Phillips, the expert who came to visit us, corroborated our suspicion that therapy was simply another type of performance. Moreover, he made a point of denouncing experts (Phillips 1997). This stage, characterized by our struggle to come to grips with the slippage of clinical authority, lasted for six months.

7   *The acephalic stage*: One day a member of our group confronted the team leader: "I'm sick and tired of you deciding everything on a whim"! The leader, who for so long questioned leadership, authority,

and experts, was rendered speechless. The pointed message from this spokesperson for the group – that the group was being run on a whim – stated clearly and logically that there was no privilege in leadership if what the leader had been saying all along was true. As though liberated, the group seized on the questioning of the group task and proceeded to discredit the leader and his ideas thus relegating him to a position of relative invisibility and depression. This stage transpired within the space of a single session.

8 *The leader survives*: The members discussed their wish to redirect the focus of the group, it would no longer concern itself with a study of performers or performance nor would the group process itself serve as data by which this research could proceed. Rather, the group task would revert back to the familiar case presentation format during which each member took a turn directing the focus of the group on individual cases and the leader was reduced to a facilitator, newly dedicated to maintaining the orderly procedure decided by the group. This stage lasted for one year until finally the leader resigned.

Case example 2

The details of this case example are all based on a laboratory group experience that is documented in a paper coauthored by one of the group participants, Dr. Arnold Rachman (1999), entitled "An Experimental Group Experience with a Silent Group Leader"; as well as conversations with the deceased group leader and coauthor, Dr. Alexander Wolf.

1 *The laboratory group*: A group of 12 psychotherapists assembled for the second half of a year-long laboratory group experience as part of an intensive training program in group therapy. The group included four women and eight men; by professional discipline, seven social workers, two psychologists, and three psychiatrists. The group was preparing for the second half of a group experience defined by the training institute as "an experimental situation ... set up to elicit and explore various interpersonal and group phenomena. The process is intended to provide a means of integrating emerging personal reactions from this group experience with basic concepts in group psychotherapy" (19). This particular group experience was to be led by guest Alexander Wolf, MD, a luminary in the world of group psychotherapy and the founder of group psychoanalysis. The group was very excited at the prospect of learning how to do psychoanalysis in groups by the founder of this technique and so they entered the experience with great expectations (see Wolf 1949–1950). The group was scheduled to meet for 15 sessions.

2   *The experiment*: The leader of the group asked the group member to consider and suggest alternate formats for the group experience rather than the focus on psychoanalysis in groups which they were expecting. The leader wanted "to do something experimental" and admitted to being "bored with doing the same old thing." Most members "apparently suppressed their resentment, disappointment, or frustration, etc. and acquiesced to the leader's request ... The will of the leader dominated over the will of the group." This planning stage covered a period of two sessions.

3   *The presentation of silence*: The third session commenced with great anticipation that the leader had decided on a proposed format. During this session, the leader remained silent for the duration of the meeting. The group engaged in trying to determine what the new format would be, not realizing that absolute silence, including some non-verbal facial communication, reflected the leader's decision.

4   *The response to silence*: Gradually,

> the group ... began to accept the reality that the leader's silence was becoming permanent ... One group of members, the smallest number, seemed to accept the leader's silence. Another subgroup of members, mostly females, was verbally and physically upset by the leader's silence. Several of them pleaded with the leader to speak. One openly wept at his unresponsiveness.
>
> Rachman and Wolf (1999, 24)

The largest subgroup of members became very angry at the leader and "encouraged the group to interact without depending on the leader's response." During this period, "several members developed plans to retaliate against the leader." This culminated in two members deciding to lock out the leader from a session. This period roughly spanned five sessions.

5   *The acephalic stage*: The members locked out the group leader from the session. For this purpose one of the members came prepared with a lock.

> The group came early to the tenth session in order to execute their plan. Eight of the twelve group members entered the group room and remained throughout the regularly scheduled session. Activity in the room consisted of laughter in besting the leader, curiosity about the leader's reaction to being locked out, anxiety about aggressing against the leader, fear of retaliation by the administration against the class, and anger for the members who did not participate ... *A sense of triumph pervaded their interaction*.
>
> 25–26 (emphasis added)

6 *The leader survives*: The leader returned and "the silent group experience lasted for four more sessions after the lock-out." This period was characterized by a flurry of inspired interpretations in an effort to account for the attempted negation of the leader. Some felt it brought the group together and "allowed a creative peer-oriented solution to the deprivation and frustration of an unresponsive leader." Others felt the group "acted-out" rather than internalize the experience as a cold rejection. Despite the force and diversity of interpretive efforts, the leader remained silent. "A sense of loss, depression, and malaise then developed in the group" (26).

Conclusion

Much can be said about the impact of the leader's silence in Case Example Two and his choice to be simultaneously absent and present (see Wolf and Schwartz 1960; Cohler, Epstein, and Issacharoff 1977). This is evidenced by author/group member Rachman's use of this experience to theorize and, in so doing, affirm and produce his and the group's psychoanalytic identity. That is, the theorizing activity of the group over the last four sessions as well as Rachman's (2003) and Rachman and Wolf (1999) published analyses that continued over years following the event, may be seen as attempts to recover the rational, productive activity of the leader that was supposed to preside over an educational experiment. This insight-oriented, rationalizing, theorizing activity stands in sharp contrast with the fleeting, irrational gleeful experience of non-productive community that revolved around the termination of the leader. The tenth session lock-out of authority was characterized by laughter, curiosity, fear, and aggression; precisely the *esprit de corps* of festival that Bataille insists is fundamental to an actual sense of community. Insofar as this experience serves no useful purpose and even entails the dissolution of personal and professional identity, it invigorates, threatens, and ultimately generates.

Likewise, Case Example 1 documents the movement of the group's destructive forces and their creative potential (for a related theoretical discussion of this group dynamic see Nitsun 1996). From the moment the IPA was established with a mandate to affirm itself and ultimately its host institution, the group proceeded to search for an object to sacrifice to this purpose (a process paralleling the mechanism described by Bataille in his anthropological depiction of the Aztecs 1991b, Volume 1). The movement toward community based on expenditure that began with an exploration of authority necessarily culminated with a confrontation of the leader in order for the group to experience community beyond any mediated, mandated, or functional purpose. While the bond of the individual group members are cemented in their united disdain and destruction of the prevailing group authority as per the "legitimate rebellion" described by Billow (2010, 120), this rebellion is not "… a strategy of social action: to modify, transform, or even overthrow the group's status quo, or adamantly to oppose its revision." Rather, the acephalic stage references a behavior that lies beyond social convention, morality, or reaction to a preestablished group task (as per Bion's sense of the group task). The liberation and play within the group was experienced in direct proportion to the loss of control and pain of the leader. In this sense the group process could be easily related to the conceptual model of "group thanatropics" as described by Kauffman (1994) in which group members realize their independence by mourning the death of the leader. Yet the acephalic stage admits of no telos nor does it revolve around any goal of redemption, its aimlessness is the quintessence of its experience as community. Again, what distinguishes Bataille's vision of an acephalic stage is its effort to conceptualize social life beyond the reductive resort to functionalism.

Finally, the survival of the leaders beyond the acephalic stage in both groups signaled the end of this brief moment of community; all that remained was a collective "sense of loss, depression, and malaise," and a return to the alternate, functionally driven productive mode. In a cyclical manner, the fleeting experience of community made possible by an acephalic stage, with all its potential for unknown and unforeseen possibilities, only recedes further with each effort to recollect, reproduce, and rationally redeem it until the next opportunity presents itself to sacrifice the authoritative structures that we hold in greatest reverence and esteem.

Bibliography

Bataille, Georges. "Program (Relative to *Acephale*)'." In *October*, 79. Edited and translated by Annette Michelson. Vol. 36, 1986/1936.

Bataille, Georges. "Base Materialism and Gnosticism." In *Visions of Excess: Selected Writings 1927–39*. Edited and translated by Allan Stoekl. Minneapolis, MN: University of Minnesota Press, 1991a/1930.

Bataille, Georges. *The Accursed Share, Vol. 1*. Translated by Robert Hurley. New York: Zone Books, 1991b/1967.

Bataille, Georges. *Acephale: Religion, Sociologie, Philosophie, 1936–1939*. Paris: Editions Jean-Michel Place, 1995 (French).

Billow, Richard M. *Resistance, Rebellion, Refusal in Groups: The 3 R's*. London: Karnac Books, 2010.

Blanchot, Maurice. *The Unavowable Community*. Translated by Pierre Joris. Barrytown, NY: Station Hill Press, 1988.

Caillois, Roger. "Brotherhoods, Orders, Secret Societies, Churches." In *The College of Sociology 1937–39*, 145–156. Edited by Denis Hollier. Translated by Betsy Wing. Minneapolis, MN: University of Minnesota Press, 1988/1938.

Canetti, Elias. *Crowds and Power*. Translated by Carol Stewart. New York: Noonday Press, 1993.

Cohler, Jonas, Lawrence Epstein, and Amnon Issacharoff. "A Psychoanalytic Evaluation of the Leader-absent or Coordinated Group Therapy Format." In *Group*, 75–89. Vol. 1 (2), 1977.

Decosta, Louise, William Buse, and Audrey Amdursky. "Personal Myths: Living Them and Pretending Them." In *Dynamic Psychotherapy*, 131–139. Vol. 4 (2), 1986.

Durkheim, Émile. *The Elementary Forms of Religious Life*. Translated by Karen E. Fields. New York: Free Press, 1995/1912.

Evans-Pritchard, E. *The Nuer*. Oxford: Clarendon Press, 1967.

Fenichel, Otto. "On Acting." In *Psychoanalytic Quarterly*, 144–160. Vol. 15, 1946.

Foucault, Michel. "A Preface to Transgression." In *Language, Counter-Memory, Practice: Selected Essays and Interviews by Michel Foucault*, 29–52. Edited by Donald F. Bouchard. Translated by Donald F. Bouchard and Sherry Simon. Ithaca, NY: Cornell University Press, 1977.

Freud, Sigmund. "Totem and Taboo." In *The Standard Edition of the Complete Psychological Works of Sigmund Freud, Volume XIII*, 1–161. Edited and translated by James Strachey. London: Hogarth Press, 1957/1912.

Galletti, Marina and Alastair Brotchie (eds). *The Sacred Conspiracy: The Internal Papers of the Secret Society of Acephale and Lectures to the College of Sociology*. Translated by Natasha Lehrer, John Harman, and Meyer Barash. London: Atlas Press, 2017.

Girard, Rene. *Violence and the Sacred*. Translated by Patrick Gregory. Baltimore, MD: Johns Hopkins University Press, 1977.

Hegarty, Paul. *Georges Bataille: Core Cultural Theorist*. London: Sage, 2000.

Heusch, Luc de. *The Drunken King, or, the Origin of the State*. Edited and translated by Roy Willis. Bloomington, IN: Indiana University Press, 1982.

Kauffman, Jeffery. "Group Thanatropics." In *Ring of Fire: Primitive Affects and Object Relations in Group Psychotherapy*, 127–147. Edited by Victor L. Schermer and Malcolm Pines. New York: Routledge, 1994.

Kristeva, Julia. *Powers of Horror: An Essay on Abjection*. Translated by Leon S. Roudiez. New York: Columbia University Press, 1982.

Mair, Lucy. *Introduction to Social Anthropology*. Oxford: Oxford University Press, 1972.

Mitchell, Andrew J. and Jason K. Winfree (eds). *The Obsessions of Georges Bataille: Community and Communication*. Albany, NY: SUNY Press, 2009.

Nancy, Jean-Luc. *The Inoperative Community*. Edited by Peter Connor. Translated by Peter Connor, Lisa Garbus, Michael Holland, and Simona Sawhney. Minneapolis, MN: University of Minnesota Press, 1991.

Nietzsche, Friedrich. *On the Genealogy of Morals: A Polemic*. Translated by Walter Kaufmann and R. J. Hollingdale. New York: Random House, 1967/1887.

Nietzsche, Friedrich. *The Will to Power*. Edited by Walter Kaufmann. Translated by Walter Kaufmann and R. J. Hollingdale. New York: Vintage Books, 1968/1901.

Nitsun, Morris. *The Anti-Group: Destructive Forces in the Group and Their Creative Potential*. New York: Routledge, 1996.

Noys, Benjamin. "Shattering the Subject: Georges Bataille and the Limits of Therapy." In *European Journal of Psychotherapy, Counseling, and Health*, 125–136. Vol. 7 (3), 2005.

Phillips, Adam. *Terrors and Experts*. Cambridge, MA: Harvard University Press, 1997.

Rachman, Arnold W. "Issues of Power, Control, and Status in Group Interaction: From Ferenczi to Foucault." In *Group*, 89–105. Vol. 27 (2/3), 2003.

Rachman, Arnold W. and Alexander Wolf. "An Experimental Group Experience with a Silent Group Leader." In *Issues: Journal of Postgraduate Center for Mental Health Group Therapy Alumni Association*, 15–31. Vol. 13, 1999.

Simmel, Georg. "The Secret Society." In *The Sociology of Georg Simmel*, 345–376. Edited and translated by Kurt H. Wolff. New York: Free Press, 1950/1908.

Wolf, Alexander. "Psychoanalysis in Groups." In *American Journal of Psychotherapy*, 16–50. Vol. 3 (4), 535–558; Vol. 4 (1), 1949–1950.

Wolf, Alexander and Emmanuel K. Schwartz. "Psychoanalysis in Groups: The Alternate Session." In *American Imago*, 101–108. Vol. 17, 1960.

Part IV

Psychotherapy with communities

Chapter 9

Triple fugue

A dialogical exploration of sovereign experience

This chapter is the result of collaboration between an anthropologist, a team of psychotherapists, and a community of artists. The impetus for this collaboration was a wish to design a counseling service for an arts conservatory that could best respond to the psychological challenges facing the aspiring performing artist in the twenty-first century. The process of constructing this service illuminated the interplay of three fields, an interaction that sustained and eventually redefined the implicit foundational ideas of performance; psychological care; and, by extension, the mission of the conservatory itself. Moreover, the inquiry into the social dynamics of this conservatory culture led to an unexpected confrontation with a pervasive institutional ethos. This underlying ethos is that of "the sovereign," whether in the experience of the artist, the psychotherapist, or the anthropologist, and especially the sovereign as an experience of personal and social transformation.

The institutional context that served as the field location for this project is The Juilliard School, located in the Lincoln Center for the Performing Arts in New York City. As of the fall of 2020, the school registered 850 undergraduate, graduate, and certificate program students. During the same period, the Counseling Service of the school consisted of a team of licensed mental health providers including ten clinical social workers, two clinical psychologists, and one psychiatrist. This paper is based on observations made over a period of 24 years by the author, the director of the Counseling Service, who is both an anthropologist and a psychoanalyst. In an effort to depict this multidisciplinary collaboration through a "transversal" narrative that privileges the relational processes of institutional culture over a static individualistic perspective (see Guattari 2000), the following text is dialogically structured as a *fugue* – a term borrowed from the culture of the institutional setting with connotations for each of the participating fields:

1   Artistically, "a fugue is a musical movement in which a definite number of parts or voices combine in stating and developing a single theme, the interest being cumulative."

Williams (1906, 114)

2   Psychologically, "The essential feature of Dissociative Fugue is sudden, unexpected, travel away from home or one's customary place of daily activities ... this is accompanied by confusion about personal identity or even the assumption of a new identity ... During a fugue, individuals generally appear to be without psychopathology and do not attract attention. At some point, the individual is brought to clinical attention, usually because of amnesia for recent events or a lack of awareness of personal identity"

American Psychiatric Association (1994), DSM-IV (481–482)

3   Anthropologically, the fugue illuminates "... an ecological niche within which mental illnesses thrive. Such niches ... provide some release that is not available elsewhere in the culture in which it thrives."

Hacking (1998, 1–2)

"Each fugue brings a different solution – in the conception of the whole form ... In the triple fugues, each theme is first developed independently (in all the voices) ... and only after that do the themes combine."

Leclaire (1998, 48)

I.

A. The artistic setting

Established in 1905, The Juilliard School today is essentially devoted to the training of performing artists in the fields of music, dance, and drama. The school is distinguished internationally by its reputation for graduating exceptional performers. Its official mission ... "is to provide the highest caliber of artistic education for gifted musicians, dancers, and actors from around the world" (Juilliard School Mission Statement 2013). Above all, the school emphasizes and expects artistic excellence. To this end, the faculty of the school consists of performers who are or have been standard bearers of artistic excellence within their respective fields. For the student, the institutional manifestation of this expectation begins with the emphasis placed on the audition for admission into the school and continues throughout the training with a series of required jury and recital performances. While academic performance makes up an important part of the curriculum, it is the evaluation and review of artistic performance – by one's teachers, peers, professional critics, and community – that are the quintessence of the Juilliard student's experience.

B. The psychotherapeutic setting

The Juilliard Counseling Service was established in 1986 as one of the first such services of its kind in a college setting let alone within a conservatory. This was entirely due to the efforts of its former president, Dr. Joseph Polisi, whose pioneering vision was to be responsive to the needs of the whole student, not simply the artist-in-training. By the time the author joined the team in 1996 the service consisted of five counselors and a psychiatrist. Their prevailing treatment model was informally psychoanalytic. From the moment of the first clinical encounter, each counselor is contending with, and greatly affected by, the personal ramifications of the institutional expectation to be extraordinary. If the pedestrian or ordinary are devalued in favor of the transcendent, what then would constitute "healing" in this rarefied clinical encounter? The empathic clinician struggling to form a provisional identification with the student's aspirations inevitably and perhaps unconsciously acquires a conviction in the "special" importance of the clinical work, a subjective experience that Lachmann has referred to as "gilt by association" (Stolorow and Lachmann 1980).Thus the entire clinical process, as an isomorph of the larger institutional expectation, easily, mutually, becomes valorized as beyond extraordinary, as sovereign. In order to understand how this experience of the sovereign implicitly defines and sanctions the treatment experience of each student, the clinician must, as always, analyze this as well. To this end, not only will the clinician explore the students' formative familial influences, but s/he must also anthropologically grasp the cultural and historical significance of the sovereign as it subtly shapes the idiom of distress that permeates the clinical encounter particular to this conservatory culture (this "transversal" approach to institutional culture foregrounds the ecological context of individual experience).

C. The sovereign

The term sovereign derives from the vulgar Latin *superanus*, eventually articulated in French as *super*, meaning above. "The spelling *–eign* which appears in the fourteenth century is due to the influence of *reign*" and finally appears as *sovereign*, meaning "a person or thing which surpasses others of the kind … Of persons: standing out above others or exceeding in some respect" as well as *sovereignty*, meaning "supremacy or pre-eminence in respect of excellence or efficacy" (Onions 1965, 1953–1954).

French social theorist Georges Bataille felt that sovereignty is best approached in economic terms; not, that is, in the usual sense of an economy based on scarcity and accumulation but rather, in the context of an unrestricted, general economy. From this perspective, all human existence, but especially sovereign existence, is made distinctive through the principle of loss, *depense*, or expenditure.

Hence the sovereign revels in the present moment, devoted to consuming, not laboring; savoring, not analyzing. This individual,

> truly enjoys the products of this world – beyond his needs. His sovereignty resides in this. Let us say that the sovereign (or the sovereign life) begins when, with the necessities ensured, the possibilities of life open up

without limit … we may call sovereign the enjoyment of possibilities that utility doesn't justify (utility being that whose end is productive activity). Life beyond utility is the domain of sovereignty.

Bataille (1991d, 198)

Bataille's economic vision focused on these so-called unproductive, un-useful activities, that is, those activities unessential for human survival that are characterized by deliberate excessive expenditure. "It is necessary to reserve the use of the word *expenditure* for the designation of these unproductive forms … they constitute a group characterized by the fact that in each case the accent is placed on a loss that must be as great as possible in order for that activity to take on its true meaning" (Bataille 1991b, 118, author's emphasis). Of particular note for the current discussion, Bataille cites "artistic production" as one among many "unproductive forms" of expenditure. He offers theater and poetry as examples of artistic expenditure and identifies poetic expression as "creation by means of loss. It's meaning therefore close to that of sacrifice" (120). Bataille further elaborates,

The poet frequently can use words only for his own loss; he is often forced to choose between the destiny of a reprobate, who is profoundly separated from society as dejecta are from apparent life, and a renunciation whose price is a mediocre activity, subordinated to vulgar and superficial needs.

120

In this view, non-productive, artistic activity affords humans the opportunity, *en masse*, to lose their preoccupation with their future, their past, their death.

What is sovereign in fact is to enjoy the present time without having anything else in view but this present time … What is the meaning of art, architecture, music, painting, or poetry if not the anticipation of a suspended, wonder-struck moment, a miraculous moment?

199–200

Approaching sovereignty through loss, Bataille will conclude that to cast off regard for history or future, utility or accumulation, and social affiliation or affirmation is to live as a sovereign: "in a fundamental sense, to live sovereignly is to escape, if not death, at least the anguish of death. Not that dying is hateful – but living servilely is hateful" (Bataille 1991d, 219). His self-styled, autoethnographic exploration of what he termed sovereign existence enabled an "inner experience" that was made possible only by his exclusion of social convention:

My inspiration is that of a sovereign existence, free of limitations of interest. I am, indeed, concerned with *being*, and being as sovereignty, with transcending the development of means – at the price, if necessary, of an impious disturbance … The issue is not that of attainment of a goal, but rather of escape from traps which goals represent.

Bataille (1989, 222)

To live a sovereign existence is to "realize the personal accomplishment of being and of its tension through concentration, through a positive asceticism, and through positive individual discipline" (Bataille 1986a, 79). Of course, Bataille's eschewing of conventional goals had personal, social ramifications. "At some point in the movement within me that refuses the servitude the human condition imposes on the multitudes, I can always stop concerning myself with other men, limiting an always precarious solidarity to my family and friends" (Bataille 2001, 188). Consequently, locating Bataille as the subject of his own relationships proved difficult for even his closest companion, who posthumously grappled with his unknowable friend:

The 'I' whose presence his search seems still to make manifest when it expresses itself, toward whom does it direct us? Certainly toward an I very different from the ego that those who knew him in the happy and unhappy particularity of life would like to evoke in the light of a memory.

Blanchot (1997, 290–291)

Solitary living, personal asceticism, and its attendant loss of fellowship, community, even one's self-experience as subject, characterized the sovereign existence for Bataille.

II.

A. The solitary artist

Behind every student performance at the Juilliard School lies several years of singular, individually focused, concentrated discipline. This might easily manifest as daily hours spent alone in a room with an inanimate instrument, memorizing scripts, composing music, or developing one's physical instrument through movement. It is not too much to say that a successful public performance implies an extraordinary amount of time spent in relative isolation. Overcoming self-consciousness and flawlessly performing is contingent on developing a bodily relationship or "muscle memory" for one's performance activity that enables effortless execution on stage. The uncanny goal of this process is an experience of decentered agency. Artistically, there is a gradual and desired sense of the performed music, lines, or movements as *flowing through* rather than *from* the performer.

This decentering experience is only intensified by the student's realization that they are surrounded by several extraordinary artists, all of whom were also singularly outstanding in their pre-Juilliard local environment. Not surprisingly, most students who enter counseling at the Juilliard Counseling Service will ultimately articulate the question of which they were initially unconscious or unaware: "Who am I doing this for; my teacher, my parents, my peers, or myself?"; this question itself being a cognate form of the developmental age-appropriate core question, "Who am I?" (Erikson 1968).

B. The solitary psychoanalyst

The Counseling Service team's psychoanalytic orientation was entirely continuous with and even structured on the model of the "private practice" that each member additionally maintained in the New York City community outside the school. Under this model all students were seen individually once weekly at a specifically set time for a 45-minute session. An essential component of this practice is the promise of non-reporting confidentiality. That is, any discussion of the student-counselor interaction with the school administration or faculty is proscribed (excepting those cases of "imminent risk involving harm to self or others" that a counselor is required by law to report). So powerful is the importance of confidentiality for the student population that a sustained effort over many years to introduce group treatment into the school culture had repeatedly failed: few if any students felt comfortable opening up in front of their peers. The resulting exclusive practice of private, confidential, individual counseling encounters was reflective, if not overtly parallel to, the individual, solitary practice underlying the students' artistic skill. As a result of their "private" practice, the counselors in the school setting occupied something of the status of "stranger" as delineated by Simmel (1950) – a liminal variant of group membership possessing "certain measures of nearness and distance" within the institution while "his position as a full-fledged member involves being outside and confronting it" (402–408). This clinical culture was contingent on the notion of solitary self-involvement and secrecy as a prerequisite to therapeutic success while inadvertently negating a social, institutional context within which all members of the community could collectively express, compare, and evaluate their individual experiences (as is the case among the Saulteaux; see Hallowell 1967).

C. Sovereignty challenged

The advent of postmodernism or "the incredulity of metanarratives" (Lyotard 1991, xxiv) has impacted the fields of anthropology, psychology, and the arts among others and has radically altered the terms by which we now understand sovereign experience. Today, anthropologists devoted to overcoming their epistemological imperialism in the ethnographic study of human interaction, home or abroad, have reimagined their discipline's task as cultural criticism (Marcus and Fischer 1986) and their participant-observation methodology as intersubjective (Rabinow 1977). The sovereign narrative authority of the ethnographer, replete with all of its ethnocentric and colonial implications, would now be decentered (Clifford 1988). Following the "linguistic turn" that precipitated postmodernism and reverberated throughout the social sciences, ethnographers sought a de-centered, relational form of participant-observation in *dialogism*, or,

> the characteristic epistemological mode of a world dominated by heteroglossia. Everything means, is understood, as part of a greater whole – there is constant interaction between meanings, all of which have the potential of conditioning others ... This dialogic imperative, mandated by the pre-existence of the language world, relative to any of its current inhabitants, insures that there can be no actual monologue.
>
> Bakhtin (1992, 426)

In a similar vein, the notion of the individual, solitary quest as represented in the life and legend of Freud had plagued the development of the psychoanalytic community for years. Several authors challenged the veracity of the myth (Sulloway 1992) or commented on the incompatibility of an individual heroic ancestor for the formation of a sustainable psychoanalytic community (Levy 2004). Moreover, the dominant one-directional orthodox Freudian model of the psychoanalyst was subverted and greatly modified by the development of relational psychoanalysis. With this new development,

> the very boundaries around the subject matter of psychoanalysis have been redrawn, and that broad reframing has had profound implications for both theory and clinical practice. *Mind has been redefined from a set of predetermined structures emerging from inside an individual organism to transactional patterns and internal structures derived from an interactive, interpersonal field"*
>
> Mitchell (1988, 17, author's emphasis)

This deconstruction of anthropological and psychoanalytic authority is ostensibly the result of progressive liberalism yet as Brown (1995) and Connolly (1993, 1994) point out, it's also simultaneously the assertion of power born of ressentiment. In this view, the new order emerges as it always has, out of negation, and is exemplified, according to Bataille, through acts of sacrifice. This sacrifice of authority and identity that had been based on a pathos of distance would inevitably be reflected in the arts as well.

III.

A. The artist as citizen

In 2005, Joseph Polisi published *The Artist as Citizen*, a book composed of speeches he had delivered over the previous 20 years of his tenure as president at Juilliard. This text clearly outlines a shift in the direction of the school's mission and training goals in response to the position of the arts entering the twenty-first century. Describing The Juilliard School he encountered in 1984 at the beginning of his presidency, Polisi states,

> there was no deep sense of community or belonging at the school ... students travelled from around the region to Lincoln Center to take their lessons, rehearse, practice, attend classes, perform, and then leave. Most of these activities were solitary in nature, and they certainly did not lend themselves to developing a sense of community.
>
> 2005, 6

Indeed, the existential tension between public, social interaction and private, individual discipline is depicted by Kogan (1989) who states,

> One must perform to get in and one must perform to make the grade there. Anxiety grabs hold and doesn't let go. All day there, one feels one should be practicing, at least to keep the level of playing up.
>
> 11

Wakin (2004) further elaborates on this dual student experience:

> Once at Juilliard, they discover the inherent paradox of being a classical musician. You are called on to be expressive, imaginative, creative, somehow in touch with the mystical reaches of art, an individual. But you are also called on to ply a craft with exceeding skill, meshing a complex of minute physical activities in the service of black markings on a page and the composers who wrote them, often submerging yourself in the crowd. And you do all this with the purpose of making a living.
>
> 9

Polisi (2005) expanded the time-honored private, individual challenges that the school was famous for by stating that "there should be no dividing line between artistic excellence and social consciousness"; he thereby asserted his "belief that artists of the twenty-first century, especially in America, must re-dedicate themselves to a broader professional agenda that reaches beyond what has been expected of them in an earlier time" (11–12). Especially important in the present context, Polisi invoked "the idea of the artist as hero" (76). Yet, as he outlines it, the terms of this new heroism will be a departure from the former individualistic, self-centered ones:

> Always stay alert to the fact that your performances are for *others*, who will be stimulated and enriched by your art. Try not to present performances in which your artistry stops abruptly at the edge of the stage. To do so will not only negate your art, but it will also rob you of the most important aspect of your profession – your ability to act as a communicator of ideas to a confused and troubled humanity.
>
> 76 (author's emphasis)

This shift in focus reverberated throughout the institution. Grimes (1993) writes, "The retooling of Juilliard has gone forward over much initial skepticism by faculty members used to operating as autonomous units and some puzzlement among music educators who see nothing wrong with the old Juilliard" (2). It remained for the Counseling Service of the school to redefine itself and its task within the new ethos that privileged the collective, the public over the private.

B. Psychotherapy socialized

In 2009, following an intensive institutional evaluation of the Juilliard Counseling Service, the school administration continued its efforts to address the previous insular character of the school's culture by literally and figuratively placing the Counseling Service on stage. The new school mandate to make counseling more openly available challenged the "ivory tower" aspect of a service built on a conservative psychoanalytic model while also confronting the stigma that faintly persisted from the twentieth century on toward psychological services in general. What had been private would now be showcased within an altered "ecological niche" that favored both a more public and more accessible service (see Siggins 2010, for a similar model of college counseling). Even the architecture of the school was radically renovated during this time, with the effect of physically opening it up to the community around it (see Figure 9.1).

It was only left now for the Counseling Service to reimagine itself. The path to a more open, communal identity would have to begin for the counselors as it does for the students, asking the same question, "Who are we doing this for?" This turnabout led to the adoption of a new focus: at any given moment the identified recipient of counseling is both the student *and* the school. Moreover, expanding the social consciousness of counseling necessarily led to a revision of how the counselors defined their clinical task: No longer would a single counselor conduct a treatment; going forward, every student was the concern of the entire counseling team thereby removing

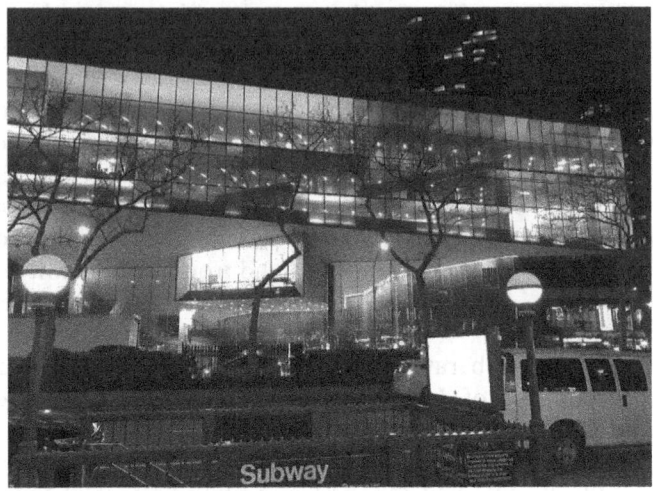

Figure 9.1 The Juilliard School (night view from the street below).
Source: Author.

any sense of sole proprietorship from the clinician. Students could pick and choose to utilize a number of different approaches available at any given time depending on their presenting circumstances. Thus clinical responsibility shifted to a team whose collective sum of knowledge is manifestly greater than its individual parts, any single member being dispensable toward the greater goal of the team. Weekly team meetings consisted of case discussions in which all members took turns presenting and "performing" their student's problems, each "performance" being understood as an unconscious enactment related to the students' familial and cultural contexts of origin; the leader identified/interpreted that derivative element of each student/counselor performance that functioned as an isomorphic expression of the idiosyncratic cultural context of the school; and the team, assuming collective responsibility for each student/ counselor dyad, mirrored back their own subjective responses in resonance with each counselor's performance, as though the treatment was their own (following the model of group dream work as designed by Ullman 1992; the relational identity construction process described by Laing 1970; and the Menominee communal treatment of schizophrenia described by Spindler 1987). Redefining the context of care as social – now including the student, the familial and cultural background of the student, the professional team context of the counselor, as well as the culture of the institution – begged a return to the question: who and what are we "healing" in the clinical encounter here today?

C. Sovereign sacrifice

According to Bataille, the sovereign authority of all social groups has been historically achieved through the expenditure of ritual sacrifice, thus underscoring his assertion that sovereignty is universally consecrated through loss (see Bataille on sacrificial behavior as it relates to the Aztec and Kwakiutl people, 1991c; to oneself, 1991d; to children, 1991e; to self-mutilation, 1991a; to erotism, 1986b; to Christianity; and to a range of non-productive behaviors, 1991b). In his own social experiment with the secret society *Acephale* that he formed "he was convinced that to bind their energies together, it was necessary to perform a human sacrifice" (Caillois 2003, 144). In this view, the sacrificial act is dynamic and transformative. Therefore, when we sacrifice an animal, "the animal dies. But the death of the animal is the becoming of consciousness" Bataille 1990, 9). Numerous anthropological accounts bear out Bataille's emphasis on the generative power of sacrifice for human social life (see de Heusch 1985; Bloch and Parry 1989; Detienne and Vernant 1989; Valeri 1985; among many others).

The corporate vitality of The Juilliard School, especially what I am terming its sovereign identity, would thus require for its sustained health and primacy, regular, ritualized, and poignant (affectively felt and meaningful) loss. However, the socioeconomic, historical, and sociocultural contexts of the school directly affect the character of this expenditure and how it is performed and represented. Where once the quasi-martyred personal sacrifice of the student could be measured in terms of the loss of social affiliation, time, and money associated with training, Polisi's vision for a more socially conscious, globally relevant Juilliard implied a less self-conscious, more socially aware commitment. By dis-privileging the narrative of the individual, private ordeal of the artist the parameters of institutional sacrifice itself were conversely expanded. Now, no aspect of the artist's life was "off-stage"; this dislocation of privacy correlated with a further diminishing of the subject.

IV.

A. The scapegoat

From van Gogh to Artaud, artists have frequently served as scapegoats – the socially venerated, sacred objects of a sacrificial expenditure that is simultaneously destructive and creative. As with all scapegoat narratives they are symbolically essential, if not actually dispensable, to that larger purpose which is the collective health of society or, in the present case, the institution. As such, scapegoating must be understood within the nuanced interactions of a dyadic social relationship. (Theories of scapegoating have highlighted this dyadic relationship in the shared identity of sacrificer and scapegoat (Mauss 1981); the transference between sacrificer and scapegoat

(Frazer 1935); "the scapegoat as vessel of vicarious atonement" (Burke 1945, 407) and "vicarious catharsis" (Becker 2005, 215); and the cathartic social healing brought about through the public persecution of the scapegoat (Girard 1987, 1989).)

This macro/micro social dialectic that implicates a scapegoat is evident at Juilliard as well. Viewed from the macro-perspective of the institution, Polisi's (2005) vision of the greater social relevance of the arts unfolded in myriad ways – from the school's expansion of its trademark name, both globally and locally, through the actual material expansion of its New York City campus building in 2009, to the establishment of a Juilliard satellite school in Tianjin, China (to commence training in the fall of 2020).

However, this ever-widening scope of institutional visibility correlated with an unexpected micro trend among its students. The demand for mental health services in the school nearly tripled between 2008 and 2019. From 2014 to 2018 the number of students registering as disabled and in need of accommodations doubled. In the same period, the number of students requesting medical leaves for psychiatric reasons tripled. Notwithstanding Conrad and Schneider's (1992, 258) observation that "the potential for medicalizing deviance has increased in the past few decades," how is this surge in the need for mental health services to be understood and what, if anything, did it have to do with the concomitant shift in artistic goals espoused by Polisi?

The students were still mandated to be extraordinary, now not only for themselves but for society. Above all, they must still, at all times, distinguish themselves from the profane or "normal." The realm of psychiatry provided the idiom by which students could distinguish themselves off-stage. Artistic performance had always been associated with social deviance or eccentricity (see Sontag 1981). Now the language of psychopathology would be adopted for the narrative reflecting the subjective response to the expanded expectation to be extraordinary. Canguilhem (1991) states "there arises in the normal man an anxiety about having remained normal, a need for disease as a test of health, that is, as its proof, an unconscious search for disease, a provocation of it" (186). We can approach this remarkable adoption of psychiatric narrative at Juilliard with the help of Sontag (1990) who suggested that suffering is precisely what we look for in the artist's work. As such, the healthy continuity of the institutional reputation for excellence is insured by evidence (or performance) of suffering. The professional role of witnessing and certifying this suffering fell to the school's counseling service.

B. The gaze

The development of medical classification as the basis for establishing deviance in the service of social authority has been well-established by Foucault (1975). In the conservatory culture specifically, where the lines between patient presentation and artistic production often blur, the clinician converts the encounter into a medical one by way of *the gaze*. This particular type of professional gaze is not passive but creative; its essence lies in the act of separating the object as organism from its subjective identity thereby establishing the category of "patient." The technical, compartmentalizing aspect of this maneuver is elucidated by Foucault (1975): "In the clinician's catalogue, the purity of the gaze is bound up with a certain silence that enables him to listen" (107); moreover, Crary (1992) notes the technical importance of "neutrality" for the development of this type of gaze as being "a condition for the formation of an observer who would be competent to consume the vast new amounts of visual imagery and information" (96).

The gaze of the silent, neutral therapist is one of total absorption. Fried (1980) identifies two important features of this rapt attention referred to as absorption. First, he describes it as a single-focused obliviousness to all else, especially the outside observer; and second, he contrasts absorption with theatricality in that the obliviousness to all others is the opposite of performance in the usual (conservatory) sense. By way of this separation, absorption intends to mark the clinical, confidential encounter as distinctly non-performative. Fried (1980) echoing Foucault, implies that absorption connotes authority within the encounter thereby attracting the non-professional outside observer into greater engagement. It is as though absorption possessed a special magic, and that its gaze created "an expanded field where a number of conceptual transformations become necessary and urgent ... concerning the question of *where the subject resides*" (Bryson 1988, 88, author's emphasis).

The conceptual transformation offered by the professional gaze finally suggests an answer to the recurring question each student and counselor asks, "who is this all for?" We saw how recent institutional developments led to self-abnegation and the resulting redefinition of subjective experience in clinical terms in the confidential space of the consulting room. During this transitional time the separation from one's own subjectivity, clinically understood as dissociation, has been desperately, increasingly expressed in the conservatory through self-laceration and suicidal ideation, all leading to an unprecedented number of hospitalizations and medical leaves. However, in a Bataillean sense, the sustained preeminence of this conservatory culture required a sacrifice for, as we have seen, sovereignty is based on loss; in this particular case, a sustained, dramatic, verifiable loss of individual subjectivity: "Sovereignty emerges as the dissolving of the subject and object worlds, and in some way represents the overcoming of the divide" (Hegarty 2000, 75).

C. Sovereignty transformed

The space where performances finally conjoin and affirm one another – the interplay of artist, clinician, and institution – is in the spectacle. Just as the separating gaze of the clinician affirms the dissociation of the artist, separation is constitutive of the spectacle. Debord (1994) comments, "Separation is the alpha and omega of the spectacle" (20); "[the spectacle's] product is separation itself" (21). Again, Fried's (1989) example may be adopted for our understanding of what is meant here by the spectacle. Fried sees absorption in the gaze of the physicians famously depicted by Thomas Eakins in his 1875 painting, *The Gross Clinic*, an absorption that is commensurate with the intense seriousness of the clinical work they are undertaking (see Figure 9.2). Subjectivity is displaced from the gazing spectator who cannot fail to be drawn in with the physicians to behold the spectacle of the sacrificed cadaver. Eakins and Fried seem to intuitively grasp that the sovereignty of the spectacle is dependent on a loss, on a requisite sacrifice – the separation of subjectivity from the object.

Debord (1994) describes in detail the sequence by which the spectator sacrifices his/her subjective sense of self:

> The spectator's alienation from and submission to the contemplated object (which is the object of his unthinking activity) works like this: the more he contemplates, the less he lives; the more readily he recognizes his own needs in the images of need proposed by the dominant system,

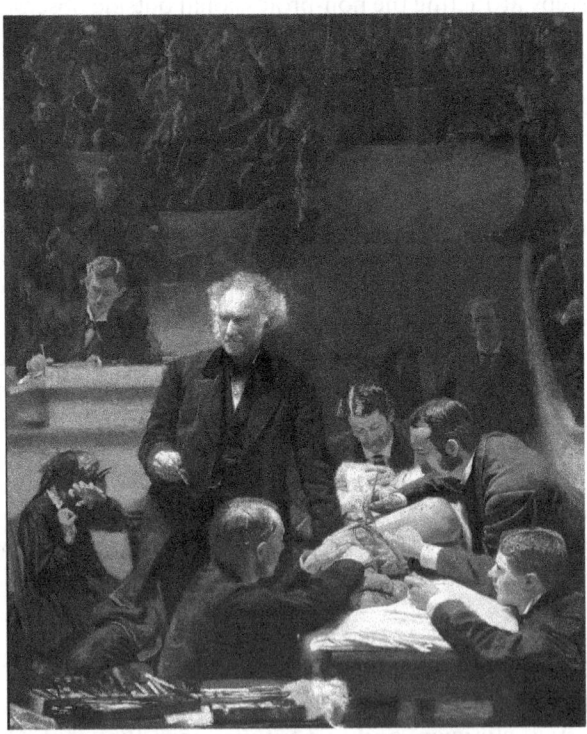

Figure 9.2 The Gross Clinic.
Source: Courtesy of Alamy, Inc.

the less he understands his own existence and his own desires. The spectacle's externality with respect to the acting subject is demonstrated by the fact that the individual's own gestures are no longer his own, but rather those of someone else who represents them to him.

23

Following Lukacs (1990), Debord regards separation as central to the alienation of the modern spectacle. To the extent that one dissociates from oneself, the spectacle attains sovereignty over individual human subjectivity.

However, according to Baudrillard (1988), even alienation implies a relationship that is lost in the postmodern transformation of the spectacle. "The private universe was certainly alienating, insofar as it separated one from others, from the world in which it acted as a protective enclosure, as an imaginary protector. Yet it also contained the symbolic benefit of alienation (the fact that the other exists) and that otherness can be played out for better or for worse ... *We no longer partake of the drama of alienation, but are in the ecstasy of communication.* And this ecstasy is obscene. Obscene is that which eliminates the gaze, the image and every representation (Baudrillard 1988, 21–22, author's emphasis). If Baudrillard is correct, it would seem that an action even more basic than separation must explain the current development of this social phenomenon by which the sovereignty of human subjectivity is completely displaced. I suggest that action is what Bataille refers to as *expenditure.*

In his ethnological examples of the Aztec and Kwakiutl societies, Bataille (1991c) refers to what may be understood as a pre-modern precursor to the spectacle – the festival. As the site of expenditure, the festival reveres

waste and destruction, as forms of excess, [as] part of the festival's essence ... One can understand how festival, representing such a paroxysm of life and contrasting so violently with the petty concerns of daily existence, seems to the individual like another world, where he feels himself sustained and transformed by powers that are beyond him.

Bataille and Caillois (1988, 281–282)

In the festival "as much energy as possible is squandered in order to produce a feeling of stupefaction" that "have no end beyond themselves" (Bataille 1991b, 118–119).

Beyond the dissociated and alienated participant of the spectacle who is estranged from him/herself, whose "gestures are no longer his own," the festival participant pursues an exuberant path toward ecstasy by deliberately losing him/herself to "intense emotions and the metamorphosis of his being" (Bataille and Caillois 1988, 282). The participant loses him/herself in the frenzy of "collective effervescence" (Durkheim 1995, 218), a structural precursor to the modern, rational dialogic form of "heteroglossia" (Bahktin

1992, 426) and, eventually, the postmodern "ecstasy of communication." This type of social expenditure is similarly alluded to by Canetti (1993) as the "discharge" of the crowd: "This is the moment when all who belong to the crowd get rid of their differences and feel equal" (17).

Bataille (1991c) elaborates on the telos particular to the festival:

> The problem posed is that of the expenditure of the surplus. We need to give away, lose, or destroy. But the gift would be senseless (and so we would never decide to give) if it did not take on the meaning of an acquisition. Hence *giving* must become *acquiring a power*. Gift-giving has the virtue of a surpassing of the subject who gives, but in exchange for the object given, the subject appropriates the surpassing: He regards his virtue, that which he had the capacity for, as an asset, as a *power* that he now possesses.
>
> 69 (author's emphases)

> By viewing man as a spender rather than as a conserver, Bataille manages to invert the usual order of economics: the moral imperative, so to speak, is the furthering of a 'good' expenditure, which we might lose sight of if we stress an inevitably selfish model of conservation or utility ... if conservation is put first, inevitably the bottled-up forces will break loose but in unforeseen, uncontrollable, and, so to speak, untheorized ways.
>
> Stoekl (2007, 38)

Rather, "we should focus our attention not on an illusory conservation, maintenance, and the steady state ... but instead on the modes of expenditure in which we, as humans, should engage" (38).

Bataille's inversion of economic life has radical implications for understanding artistic expression, the goal of an arts conservatory, and the counseling role within it. Whether intentionally or not, Polisi pushed the school in the only direction that would assure its sovereign reputation in a world fixed on accumulation and utility. This is all the more remarkable (if not ironic) in the context of a conservatory devoted to the conservation and preservation of the "classical" performing arts. He was prescient in his belief that the narcissistic preoccupation with one's own artistic production could be insufficient to qualify as extraordinary in an increasingly acquisitive and conservative society. The Juilliard spectacle is measured by more than artistic excellence; it's measured in the willingness of the school to spend its dearest resource by committing its students to a goal "that reaches beyond what has been expected of them in an earlier time" (Polisi 2005, 12). With this mandate in mind, the school's counselors have become midwives to a "good" expenditure through their reinterpretation of loss and dissociation as a transcendent "surpassing of the subject" (Bataille 1991c, 69) as well as their renewed understanding of separation, following Bataille (1991a, 67, author's emphasis), as "the necessity of throwing oneself or something of oneself *out of oneself*" – the sublime prerequisite to sovereign experience.

Bibliography

American Psychiatric Association. *Diagnostic and Statistical Manual of Mental Disorders, 4th Edition.* Washington, DC: American Psychiatric Association, 1994.

Bakhtin, Mikhail, M. *The Dialogic Imagination.* Edited by Michael Holquist. Translated by Caryl Emerson and Michael Holquist. Austin, TX: University of Texas Press, 1992.

Bataille, Georges. "Program (Relative to Acephale)." In *Georges Bataille: Writings on Laughter, Sacrifice, Nietzsche, Un-knowing,* 79. Translated by Annette Michelson. In *October.* Vol. 36, 79 Spring, 1986a/1936.

Bataille, Georges. *Erotism: Death & Sensuality.* Translated by Mary Dalwood. San Francisco, CA: City Lights Books, 1986b.

Bataille Georges. "Autobiographical Note." In *My Mother, Madame Edwards, The Dead Man,* 215–222. Translated by Austryn Wainhouse. New York: Marian Boyars, 1989.

Bataille, Georges. "Hegel, Death and Sacrifice." In *On Bataille,* 9–28. Edited by Alan Stoekl. Translated by Jonathan Strauss. New Haven, CT: Yale French Studies. Vol. 78, 1990/1955.

Bataille, Georges. "Sacred Mutilation and the Severed Ear of Vincent Van Gogh." In *Visions of Excess: Selected Writings, 1927–1939,* 61–72. Edited and translated by Alan Stoekl. Minneapolis, MN: University of Minnesota Press, 1991a/1930.

Bataille Georges. "The Notion of Expenditure." In *Visions of Excess: Selected Writings, 1927–1939,* 116–129. Edited and translated by Alan Stoekl. Minneapolis, MN: University of Minnesota Press, 1991b/1933.

Bataille, Georges. *The Accursed Share, Vol. I.* Translated by Robert Hurley. New York: Zone Books, 1991c/1967.

Bataille Georges. "Sovereignty." In *The Accursed Share, Vol. III,* 197–430. Edited by author Georges Bataille. Translated by Robert Hurley. New York: Zone Books, 1991d/1976.

Bataille, Georges. *The Trial of Gilles de Rais.* Translated by Richard Robinson. Los Angeles, CA: Amok Books, 1991e.

Bataille Georges. *The Unfinished System of Knowledge.* Edited by Stuart Kendall. Translated by Michelle Kendall and Stuart Kendall. Minneapolis, MN: University of Minnesota Press, 2001.

Bataille, Georges and Caillois, Roger. "Festival." In *The College of Sociology, 1937–39,* 279–303. Edited by Denis Hollier. Translated by Betsy Wing. Minneapolis, MN: University of Minnesota Press, 1988/1939.

Baudrillard, Jean. *The Ecstasy of Communication.* Translated by Bernard and Caroline Schutze. Edited by Sylvere Lotringer. New York: Semiotext(e), 1988.

Becker, Ernest. *The Earnest Becker Reader.* Edited by Daniel Liechty. Seattle, WA: University of Washington Press, 2005.

Blanchot, Maurice. *Friendship.* Translated by Elizabeth Rottenberg. Stanford, CA: Stanford University Press, 1997/1971.

Bloch, Maurice and Jonathan Parry (eds). *Death and the Regeneration of Life.* Cambridge: Cambridge University Press, 1989.

Brown, Wendy. *States of Injury: Power and Freedom in Late Modernity.* Princeton, NJ: Princeton University Press, 1995.

Bryson, Norman. "The Gaze in the Expanded Field." In *Vision and Visuality*, 87–114. Edited by Hal Foster. Seattle, WA: Bay Press, 1988.

Burke, Kenneth. *A Grammar of Motives.* New York: Prentice-Hall, 1945.

Caillois, Roger. "Interview with Gilles Lapouge, June, 1970." In *The Edge of Surrealism: A Roger Caillois Reader*, 141–146. Edited by Claudine Frank. Translated by Claudine Frank and Camille Naish. Durham, NC: Duke University Press, 2003/1970.

Canguilhem, Georges. *The Normal and the Pathological.* Translated by Carolyn R. Fawcett. New York: Zone Books, 1991/1966.

Canetti, Elias. *Crowds and Power.* Translated by Carol Stewart. New York: Noonday Press. 1993.

Clifford, James. "On Ethnographic Authority." In *The Predicament of Culture: Twentieth-Century Ethnography, Literature, and Art*, 21–54. Edited by James Clifford. Cambridge, MA: Harvard University Press, 1988.

Connolly, William. E. *Political Theory and Modernity.* Ithaca, NY: Cornell University Press, 1993.

Connolly, William. E. *Identity/Difference: Democratic Negotiations of Political Paradox.* Ithaca, NY: Cornell University Press, 1994.

Conrad, Peter and Joseph W. Schneider. *Deviance and Medicalization: From Badness to Sickness.* Philadelphia, PA: Temple University Press, 1992.

Crary, Jonathan. *Techniques of the Observer: On Vision and Modernity in the Nineteenth Century.* Cambridge, MA: MIT Press, 1992.

Debord, Guy. *The Society of the Spectacle.* Translated by Donald. Nicholson-Smith. New York: Zone Books, 1994/1967.

Detienne, Marcel. and Jean-Pierre Vernant. *The Cuisine of Sacrifice among the Greeks.* Translated by Paula Wissing. Chicago, IL: The University of Chicago Press, 1989.

Durkheim, Émile. *The Elementary Forms of Religious Life.* Translated by Karen E. Fields. New York: Free Press, 1995/1912.

Eakins, Thomas. *The Gross Clinic.* Courtesy of Alamy, Inc, 1875.

Erikson, Erik. *Identity, Youth, and Crisis.* New York: Norton, 1968.

Foucault, Michel. *The Birth of the Clinic: An Archaeology of Medical Perception.* Translated by A. M. Sheridan Smith. New York: Viking Books, 1975.

Frazer, James G. *The Golden Bough: A Study in Magic and Religion, Volume VI: The Scapegoat.* New York: Macmillan Company, 1935.

Fried, Michael. "The Primacy of Absorption." In *Absorption and Theatricality: Painter and Beholder in the Theater of Diderot*, 7–70. Edited by Michael Fried. Berkeley, CA: University of California Press, 1980.

Fried, Michael. *Realism, Writing, Disfiguration.* Chicago, IL: The University of Chicago Press, 1989.

Girard, Rene. "Generative Scapegoating." In *Violent Origins: Ritual Killing and Cultural Formation*, 73–105. Edited by Robert G. Hamerton-Kelly. Stanford, CA: Stanford University Press, 1987.

Girard, Rene. *The Scapegoat*. Translated by Yvonne Freccero. Baltimore, MD: Johns Hopkins University Press, 1989.

Grimes, William. "Too Many Musicians? An Overhaul at Juilliard – A Special Report; A New Juilliard for a More Challenging Era." In *The New York Times*, June 2, 1993. Retrieved from www.nytimes.com/1993/06/02/arts/too-many-musicians-overhaul-juilliard-special-report-new-juilliard-for-more.html.

Guattari, Felix. *The Three Ecologies*. Translated by Ian Pindar and Paul Sutton. New Brunswick: Athlone Press, 2000.

Hacking, Ian. *Mad Travelers: Reflections on the Reality of Transient Mental Illness*, Charlottesville, VA: University Press of Virginia, 1998.

Hallowell, Alfred Irving. "The Social Function of Anxiety in a Primitive Society." In *Culture and Experience*, 266–275. Edited by A. I. Hallowell. Philadelphia, PA: University of Pennsylvania Press, 1967.

Hegarty, Paul. *Georges Bataille: Core Cultural Theorist*. London: Sage Publications, 2000.

Heusch, Luc de. *Sacrifice in Africa: A Structuralist Approach*. Translated by Linda O'Brien and Alice Morton.Bloomington, IN: Indiana University Press, 1985.

Juilliard School Mission Statement, 2013. Retrieved from www.juilliard.edu.

Kogan, Judith. *Nothing but the Best: The Struggle for Perfection at the Juilliard School*. New York: Limelight Editions, 1989.

Laing, Ronald D. *The Divided Self: An Existential Study in Sanity and Madness*. Baltimore, MD: Penguin Books, 1970.

Leclaire, Serge. *A Child is being Killed: On Primary Narcissism and the Death Drive*. Translated by Marie-Claude Hays. Stanford, CA: Stanford University Press, 1998.

Levy, Stephen. "Splendid Isolation." In *Journal of the American Psychoanalytic Association*, 971–973. Vol. 52 (4), 2004.

Lukacs, Georg. *History and Class Consciousness: Studies in Marxist Dialectics*. Cambridge, MA: MIT Press, 1990/1968.

Lyotard, Jean-Francois. *The Postmodern Condition: A Report on Knowledge*. Minneapolis, MN: University of Minnesota Press, 1991.

Marcus, George and Michael M. J. Fischer. *Anthropology as Cultural Critique: The Experimental Moment in the Human Sciences*. Chicago, IL: The University of Chicago Press, 1986.

Mauss, Marcel and Henri Hubert. *Sacrifice: Its Nature and Functions*. Translated by W. D. Halls. Chicago, IL: The University of Chicago Press, 1981/1898.

Mitchell, Stephen. *Relational Concepts in Psychoanalysis: An Integration*. Cambridge, MA: Harvard University Press, 1988.

Onions, Charles Talbot (ed.). *The Shorter Oxford English Dictionary of Historical Principles*. London: Oxford University Press, 1965.

Polisi, Joseph W. *The Artist as Citizen*. Pompton Plains, NJ: Amadeus Press, 2005.

Rabinow, Paul. *Reflections on Fieldwork in Morocco*. Berkeley, CA: University of California Press, 1977.

Siggins, Lorraine D. "Working with the Campus Community." In *Mental Health Care in the College Community*, 143–155. Edited by Jerald Kay and Victor Schwartz. Hoboken, NJ: John Wiley & Sons, 2010.

Simmel, Georg. "The Stranger." In *The Sociology of Georg Simmel*, 402–408. Edited and translated by Kurt H. Wolff. New York: Free Press, 1950/1908.

Sontag, Susan. *Under the Sign of Saturn*. New York: Vintage Books, 1981.

Sontag, Susan. "The Artist as Exemplary Sufferer." In *Against Interpretation and Other Essays*, 39–48. Edited by Susan Sontag. New York: Anchor Books, 1990.

Spindler, George. "Joe Nepah, a 'Schizophrenic' Menominee Peyotist." In *The Journal of Psychoanalytic Anthropology: A Quarterly Journal of Culture and Personality*, 1–16. Vol. 10 (1), 1987.

Stoekl, Allan. *Bataille's Peak: Energy, Religion, and Postsustainability*. Minneapolis, MN: University of Minnesota Press, 2007.

Stolorow, Robert and Frank Lachmann. *Psychoanalysis of Developmental Arrests: Theory and Treatment*. New York: International Universities Press, 1980.

Sulloway, Frank. *Freud: Biologist of the Mind*. Cambridge, MA: Harvard University Press, 1992.

Ullman, Montague. *Appreciating Dreams: A Group Approach*. London: Sage Publications, 1992.

Valeri, Valerio. *Kingship and Sacrifice: Ritual and Society in Ancient Hawaii*. Translated by Paula Wissing. Chicago, IL: The University of Chicago Press, 1985.

Wakin, Daniel J. "The Juilliard Effect: Ten Years Later." In *The New York Times*, December 12, 2004. Retrieved from www.nytimes.com/2004/12/12/arts/music/the-juilliard-effect-ten-years-later.html.

Williams, Vaughn R. "Fugue." In *Grove's Dictionary of Music and Musicians, Volume 2*, 9–20. Edited by John Alexander Fuller Maitland. New York: Macmillan, 1906.

Part V

The end(s) of psychotherapy

Chapter 10

Do no harm/please harm me

This is the story of a storyteller (Figure 10.1). Do we still even recognize this dying art? To be sure, we begin with this description by Walter Benjamin (2002) that portrays the practice as it disappears:

> Familiar though his name may be to us, the storyteller is by no means a force today. He has already become something remote from us and is moving further away ... One meets with fewer and fewer people who know how to tell a tale properly ... One reason for this phenomenon is obvious: experience has fallen in value (143) ... Every morning brings

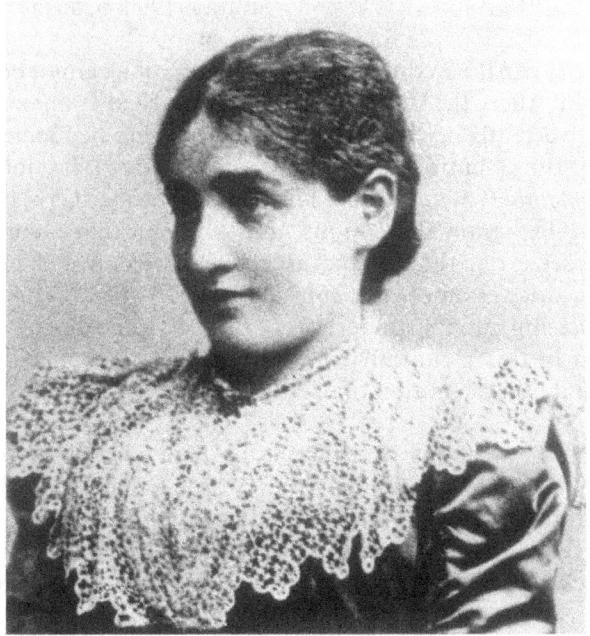

Figure 10.1 Anna O.
Source: Courtesy of Alamy, Inc.

us news from across the globe, yet we are poor in noteworthy stories. This is because nowadays no event comes to us without already being shot through with explanations. In other words, by now almost nothing that happens benefits storytelling; almost everything benefits information. Actually, it is half the art of storytelling to keep a story free from explanation as one recounts it ... The most extraordinary things, marvelous things, are related with the greatest accuracy, but the psychological connections among the events are not forced on the reader. It is left up to him to interpret things the way he understands them, and thus the narrative achieves an amplitude that information lacks ... the more natural the process by which the storyteller forgoes psychological shading, the greater becomes the story's claim to a place in the memory of the listener.

147–149

We can extend Benjamin's critique further by equating what he refers to as "information" with "content":

Whatever it may have been in the past, the idea of content is today mainly a hindrance, a nuisance, a subtle or not so subtle philistinism [and] what the overemphasis on the idea of content entails is the perennial, never consummated project of *interpretation*.

Sontag (1990, 5, author's emphasis)

If, indeed, a story can have content, then interpretation cannot be far behind, even to the point where the story itself may be regarded as an interpretation. Benjamin inadvertently speaks to this function where he identifies what he feels is "one of the essential features of every real story: it contains openly or covertly, *something useful*" (2002, 145, emphasis added). Yet here we must depart, despite Benjamin's intentions, into a region that Georges Bataille was quick to seize on, that is, the exceptional circumstances where the usefulness of a story is simply not apparent.

Before wandering into the modern story of how the field of psychoanalysis was conceived in this lacuna in "usefulness," we are obliged to consider Bataille's thought on the notion of usefulness itself; he states,

Every time the meaning of a discussion depends on the fundamental value of the word *useful* – in other words, every time the essential question touching on the life of human societies is raised, no matter who intervenes and what opinions are expressed – it is possible to affirm that the debate is necessarily warped and that the fundamental question is eluded.

Bataille (1991b, 116, author's emphasis)

Rather, as an alternative to "useful" storytelling, Bataille would hint at a simple, amoral, and non-useful mimetic character of storytelling: in his words,

> It is clear that the world is purely parodic, in other words, that each thing seen is the parody of another, or is the same thing in a deceptive form ... Everyone is aware that life is parodic and that it lacks an interpretation.
>
> Bataille (1991c, 5)

Storytelling, as "writing, for Georges Bataille, doubles as experience. No longer, or not merely, the representation of 'some occasion', some ecstatic embrace in the woods, writing itself performs the experience of loss, performs ecstasy" (Botting and Wilson 1993, 195).

I am suggesting that the birth of psychoanalysis from the phantom pregnancy of Anna O. follows from just such an ecstatic notion of storytelling, and that her storytelling has mimetically reverberated for nearly 140 years, spawning various and sustaining versions of an origin myth. Moreover, this myth possesses a peculiar, defining character. Addressing the story of Anna O., Ellenberger (1993) decries the "deficiencies [that] lead inevitably to the formation of historical myths, and it is by this means that certain domains of the history of psychiatry have come to be obscured by a thick cloud of legend" (254–255). Indeed, there is no end to the efforts to point out the "deficiencies" of Anna O.'s treatment and the record of it as a prelude to telling the "real" story. An explanation is offered by psychoanalytic scholar Pollock (1984):

> So when we have a patient who is well known in the community, and we have a therapist who is well known in the community, and we have a reluctance to go ahead and acknowledge certain facts, it may well be that there are certain kinds of omissions and certain kinds of distortions which should be handled in other ways.
>
> 29

This literature of qualifications, apologias, and competing interpretations is acknowledged and then predictably reinforced by Maroda (2010):

> Why are there so many distortions and misrepresentations in the case of Anna O., and why are they important? The answer to these questions lies in the multiple issues surrounding the treatment itself, including those centered on the case report created by Breuer and Freud – both what was included and what was excluded.
>
> 678

The activity of interpretation, the *sine qua non* of the psychoanalytic project, derives impetus from these never-ending, "never consummated" efforts to get to the bottom of what Anna O. was all about. Newly recovered historical "content" has been heralded as holding the key (Forrester and Cameron 1999). Yet I am proposing a reconsideration of this quest for historical and psychological accuracy as a vital aspect of the myth. Perhaps a focus on the most compelling interpretation as well as the historical veracity of clinical data are less important than the myth-making project itself. Indeed, the starting point for many efforts toward the "correct" interpretation of Anna O.'s experience begins with the assertion that the famous case report about her, published by Freud and Breuer (1957) "must be regarded as largely confabulated" (Shorter 1997, 23). Borch-Jacobsen (1996, 10) states, "Paradoxically enough, the very myth that forms the basis of our modern belief in the redemptive value of recollection and narration has stubbornly resisted historicization. Everyone knows perfectly well that the cure of Anna O. is a myth."

Suppose then we were to revisit the Anna O. story as a story about a woman who told and enacted stories that were remarkably distinguished in their ability to generate more enactments and more stories; as an origin myth drawn from the ecstatic (otherwise derided as hysterical) experiences of a modern day Sibyl who, like the Sybil of antiquity "addresses God [in the figure of Breuer] and appeals to him to release her from prophetic ecstasy" (Parke 1988, 9); and who possessed the enigmatic talent to conceive and endlessly regenerate an entire human project that would be destined (cursed?) to repeatedly try and fail at interpreting the circumstances of its own origin. This, then, is the story of,

> how the hysteric, reported to be incurable, sometimes – and more and more often – took the role of the resistant heroine: the one whom psychoanalytic treatment would never be able to reduce. The one who roused Freud's passion through the spectacle of femininity in crisis, and the one, the only one, who knew how to escape him. (*This version of hysterical history is, indeed, what keeps the very history of psychoanalysis going.*)
> Cixous and Clement (1986, 9, emphasis added)

Our story will necessarily be polyphonic with respect to the multiple genres and inventive tropes of interpretation invoked in her wake. However, at the outset and in the midst of this cacophony of commentaries we begin with Anna O. herself; although she was "often written about, she was rarely permitted to speak on her own behalf" (Gillman 2008, 7). She is quoted as stating presciently, emphatically, "With respect to works of art and to people which one can only 'truly appreciate' or 'understand' when annotated, I am very suspicious, I advise you to be also" (in Guttman 2001, 1). I read this as her mistrust of precisely the "explanations" that Benjamin cited as being inimical to storytelling. Her warning notwithstanding, we are tempted to contextualize the circumstances of her story.

Possibilities for being heard, let alone any type of achievement for a woman of her time, were blatantly restricted; "in Central European culture of the nineteenth century ... one entered into polite society through the reading (and perhaps also the writing) of literature" (8). Hence, the recourse for a woman seeking attention would be through the arts or as an object of medical interest, or, specifically in Anna O.'s case, her writing or her symptomology.

> In Vienna, as elsewhere, [the concept of dramatic catharsis] was discussed among scholars and in the salons and even assumed for a time the proportions of a craze ... It seems very possible that an intelligent girl like Anna O. might have acquainted herself with the subject and have unconsciously incorporated this knowledge into the dramatic plot of her illness.
>
> Sulloway (1992, 56–57)

Her family, originally from Eastern Europe, "had never really left this atmosphere of puritanical inhibition, although they moved to Vienna" (Shorter 1997, 33). This resulted in a certain anxiety of influence within Anna O.'s home with parental over-protectiveness fueling a restlessness not unusual for a first-generation child confronting the urban pull of assimilation. Perhaps it is for this reason that Anna O. is often perceived as having been both precocious and naïve. However, there is another strain of historical scholarship that portrays Anna O. as possessing agency, even to the point of being creatively manipulative. Being that this side of Anna O. is predicated on a knowledge of her famous encounter with the fledgling field of psychoanalysis, let's first consider that feature of her story for which she is most widely known.

Historian of psychiatry Henri Ellenburger (1993) provides a typical and widely accepted summation of the Anna O. legend:

> To this day, the most elementary account of psychoanalysis begins with the story of a mysterious young woman, 'Anna O.', whose numerous hysterical symptoms disappeared one by one as Josef Breuer was able to make her evoke the specific circumstances that had led to their appearance. The patient herself called this procedure 'the talking cure' or 'chimney-sweeping,' while Breuer called it 'catharsis.' Anna O.'s treatment took place from 1880 to 1882, but the case history was published only thirteen years later, that is, in 1895, in Breuer's and Freud's *Studies on Hysteria*. From that time on, Anna O.'s story has been cited as the prototype of a cathartic cure and as one of the basic occurrences that led Freud to the creation of psychoanalysis.
>
> 255–256

This encounter between Drs. Breuer and Freud, known to us through the storytelling of their case studies in *Studies on Hysteria* (1895) which featured a novel treatment of hysteria, and Anna O., a young woman whose verbal and behavioral restrictions and inhibitions limited her initial storytelling to non-verbal affects and bodily expression, proved pivotal. Through their collaboration, the first of its kind, psychoanalysis came to "be seen as a translation into theory of the language of hysteria" (Hunter 1983, 485). Viewed more critically, Carson (1994, 29) states,

> Freud and Breuer claim, the symptoms disappear – cleansed by the simple cathartic ritual of draining off the bad sound of unspeakable things … As if the entire female gender were a kind of collective bad memory of unspeakable things, patriarchal order like a well-intentioned psychoanalyst, seems to conceive its therapeutic responsibility as the channeling of this bad sound into politically appropriate containers.

We are left with Anna O. as the reluctant heroine recruited and exploited by the psychoanalytic project that then deemed her their founding collaborator. Breuer's and Freud's story, and her place in it, was "useful" for them. However, this was evidently not useful for her, for the remainder of her life Anna O. barely acknowledged or discussed her role as the mother of "the talking cure."

Yet this view of Anna O. as the unwitting representative victim of Victorian patriarchal oppression is incomplete. Returning to the aforementioned, alternative perspective that allows for her agency and creative innovation within a sexually restrictive cultural era, Anna O. seized the opportunity provided by the arrival of these professional figures from outside her home. Shorter (1997, 24) states, "What previous scholars have not fully perceived in these events is how this unhappy young woman could manipulate the climate of anxious hypochondriasis that pervaded the culture she inhabited" [and that this] "climate of anxious hypochondriasis that characterized the Jews of Eastern Europe ensured that others were vulnerable to such manipulation" (33).

> … To what extent did she consciously produce these symptoms? The more conscious the process, the more her main diagnosis shifts toward simulation and away from hysteria, which entails a presumably unconscious process … Breuer, transfixed in the headlights of the illness, was more a victim of this young patient than he was the innovator of 'dynamic psychological treatment'.
>
> 30

Indeed, Lacan (2018, 51) echoes this sentiment regarding Anna O.'s impact on her doctors,

> There was a certain Anna O. who knew a thing or two about the maneuver of the hysteric's game. She presented all of her little story,

all her fantasies, to Herren Breuer and Freud, who leapt on them like little fish into water ... Anna O. had him quite perfectly, Freud himself, in her sights. But he was clearly a bit harder to take in than the other fellow, Breuer.

Moreover, Hunter (1983, 475) notes, "After her conversion symptoms had ceased, and while she was passing through what Breuer called a temporary depression, [Anna O.] told him that 'the whole thing had been simulated'." "In fact, Anna O. represented a quite ordinary case of somatization combined with a not inconsiderable measure of *playacting*" (Shorter 1997, 24, emphasis added).

When considering the latter portrait of a canny and creative Anna O., it seems that the notion of mimetic play might more accurately reflect what it is that we think we know of her. By mimetic play I refer to a general process by which "the imitator – *mimetes* – that is to say the creative as well as the executive artist, knows not himself whether the thing he imitates is good or bad; mimesis is mere play to him, not serious work" (Huizinga 1955, 162, author's emphasis). Caillois (2001) further elaborates on this play of mimicry:

> Play can consist not only of deploying actions or submitting to one's fate in an imaginary milieu, but of becoming an illusory character oneself, and of so behaving. One is thus confronted with a diverse series of manifestations, the common element of which is that the subject makes believe or makes others believe that he is someone other than himself. He forgets, disguises, or temporarily sheds his personality in order to feign another. I prefer to designate these phenomena by the term mimicry (19) ... Mimicry consists in deliberate impersonation, which may readily become a work of art, contrivance, or cunning. The actor must work out his role and create a dramatic illusion.
>
> 77–78

I would suggest that beyond her reputation as the woman who pioneered the novel treatment based on *catharsis*, Anna O. would more correctly be regarded as the woman who found a way to survive her circumstances through the play of *mimesis*. Moreover, I believe that both the details of her treatment as well as her life beyond the treatment support this conclusion. Even the quintessential feature of the psychoanalytic legend, in which Anna O. is given over to cathartic experience in the throes of a hypnotic trance, may alternatively be considered through the lens of a mimetic process. Borch-Jacobsen (1993, 110, author's emphasis) explains,

> The possessed person, *who no longer speaks*, really is asked, in the course of the trance, to name the spirit and the malefic power that haunts him. But in what form? In the form of the mimetic speech in which the

possessed person vaticinates, as Plato said about the poet-mimetician, 'under the name of the other.' Hence this speech is not a speech of dialogue (with the spirit, with others in general); rather it is a matter of inspired speech in which the 'self' is indistinguishable from the 'other' (even if, from the doctor's point of view and from that of the assembled spectators, it serves to put an end to that pathetic identification). By privileging the role of speech in the trance, we consequently risk forgetting its very particular character, which is to indicate an experience that is lived outside of representation, and which, by this very fact, can be communicated, *in language*, only in the form of the mimetic indistinction between 'self' and 'other'.

Borch-Jacobsen's reference to the "inspired speech" of mimesis returns us to that storytelling that is ecstatic, that is parodic, and that serves no useful purpose. Mimetic play is parodic in the sense that "parody is where mimicry exposes construction" (Taussig 1993, 68), in this case the construction of the psychoanalytic project. Consequently, what appears to be Breuer's discovery is actually Anna O.'s invention, or rather, her innovative, improvised enactment of what she understood her expected role in this new game to be. This playful process is captured with intuitive brilliance by R. D. Laing (1970, 28) where he states, "The behavior of the patient is to some extent a function of the behavior of the psychiatrist in the same behavioral field. The standard psychiatric patient is a function of the standard psychiatrist." Thus, Anna O. remains a reflection (and retains the potency) of whoever conjures her for whatever purpose.

   Anna O. was born on February 27, 1859. After her father was made wealthy through an inheritance, her family, of Eastern European roots, relocated to Vienna. "I led the usual life of a girl of the middle class" is how she referred to herself (Edinger 1968, 14).

[Her] typical day probably began with a horseback ride with friends. Since [her family] had servants for the major care of the house, the rest of the day was devoted to light household chores – tatting lace, sewing, stringing pearls, embroidering. These crafts were considered appropriate, decorative activities for women. She also read passionately, showing a particular love of Shakespeare. She played the piano but never attained the level of skill she desired. The loving-kindness of her character, combined with an instilled sense of duty, often led her to do charitable work for poor Jews living in other districts. In the evenings ... formally attired, she might attend a concert, the theater, or a party, all activities of which she was passionately fond. Expectations of her were small and superficial: She was to prepare herself for entry into high society by dressing in the latest fashion, attending tea parties, and learning the nuances of politesse. She moved easily in her social circle, and her gaiety and charm seemed to enchant everyone who met her ... [In the summer, in the countryside, she] whiled the days swimming, boating, hiking, and daydreaming during walks in nearby meadows.

Guttmann (2001, 39)

Regarding play, particularly sexual play, Anna O.,

probably had the same seductive, charming, vivacious qualities as a little girl that she possessed as an adult ... Dr. Edinger [her close friend] described her as 'very seductive' with men, saying she could 'twist a man around her fingers if she wanted to.'

Freeman (1972, 244)

"In a group of men, she was absolutely bewitching. I've seen her easily beguile them. She had many admirers; without doubt they'd all ask for her hand in marriage. Even elderly, she must have been very seductive for men" (quote from Edinger in Safouan 1987, 51). Freud, himself, wrote to his fiancée Martha Bernays (herself a close friend of Anna O.), that a colleague of his "is completely enchanted by the girl, by her provocative appearance in spite of her gray hair, by her wit and cleverness," to which Martha responded,

It is curious that no man other than her physician of the moment got close to poor [Anna O.], that is, when she was healthy she already had the power to turn the heads of the most sensible of men.

Forrester (1994, 19)

Yet "in spite of the daring she showed in many respects, sexually [she] was an extremely inhibited woman" (Freeman 1972, 246).

Her sexual conservatism was at least partially attributable to her deep Orthodox Jewish upbringing.

[Her] education consisted of both religious and secular training. As a daughter in an orthodox family she received basic religious training. She knew both Hebrew and Yiddish, prayers and rituals of the Jewish calendar, rules for keeping an orthodox Jewish kitchen, laws related to the preparation of food, and ritual menstrual hygiene. However, as a woman she did not receive any formal religious education in Jewish laws and traditions ... On leaving school at 16 she was fluent in English, French, and Italian. There were, however, no further educational opportunities open to her or indeed any woman in Vienna at this time. She stayed at home living the life of a middle-class daughter of marriageable age, which consisted of riding, walks, tea parties, theater, concerts, sewing, and needlework for one's trousseau, and precious little stimulation.

Kimball (2000, 21)

Her exceptional conservatism was additionally due to the fact that "she was raised with great protectiveness and had no contact with boys" (Shorter 1997, 24); and also partially due to the cautiousness of her parents following the death of both of Anna O's sisters during her childhood. Perhaps most importantly, though, her consuming devotion to her father with whom she shared a very close relationship is felt to have also contributed to her noticeable lack of interest in ideas of sex, dating, and romance that would have been typical of a woman her age in her time and place (Freeman 1972).

By all accounts the cumulative impact of this lifestyle resulted in insufferable boredom for Anna O. as she entered early adulthood. However, as Benjamin (2002, 149) notes in his reflection on storytelling, "boredom is the apogee of mental relaxation. Boredom is the dream bird that hatches the egg of experience" and, as such, serves as the precondition needed for the ambience of storytelling and listening. Accordingly,

> This brought Anna O. to escape from her daily domestic situation into long daydreams that she was in the habit of calling her 'private theater.' However these daydreams did not interfere with her daily activities, and other family members were not aware of them.
>
> Ellenberger (1993, 256)

Perhaps one of the reasons Anna O.'s private world eluded the attention of her family was that her father was slowly dying of tuberculosis in the same house. Anna O. was often nursing him for extended periods of time as he deteriorated. The selflessness required of this young adult would have been great. Indeed, it is commonly presumed that her emotional neglect combined with the burden of caring for her father, and the prospect of losing yet another family member could all have contributed to the development of symptoms for which she would finally receive extraordinary attention.

> In connection with the psychic stress of nursing, Anna O. began to develop some hysterical symptoms of both a motor and a sensory variety ... All these symptoms unfolded themselves over the period of July to December 1880, and are quite unremarkable in that they represent the typical 'marketbasket' of hysteria of the day, the kinds of symptoms the culture had told young nineteenth-century woman they must develop if they wished to be considered 'ill'.
>
> Shorter (1997, 25)

In the fall of 1880, when Dr. Josef Breuer was called by the family to examine Anna O., "she was twenty-one years old, beautiful, petite, 4'11", with dark hair and sparkling blue eyes" (Guttmann 2001, 21). Breuer, most likely the family physician and already highly esteemed in Vienna, was contacted on account of her unremitting cough. He reports his initial impressions:

> She was markedly intelligent, with an astonishingly quick grasp of things and penetrating intuition. She possessed a powerful intellect which would have been capable of digesting solid mental pabulum and which stood in need of it – though without receiving it after she had left school. She had great poetic and imaginative gifts, which were under the control of a sharp and critical common sense ... Her will-power was energetic, tenacious and persistent; sometimes it reached the pitch of an obstinacy which only gave way out of kindness and regard for other people.
>
> Breuer and Freud (1957, 21)

From the outset and throughout the case, we are constantly confronted with a peculiar, idiosyncratic trait, that is, Anna O.'s pervasive splitting, doubling, twinning, and a host of other occurrences in duplicate. Her preponderance of pairing is eventually attributed by the two doctors, Breuer and Freud, to processes of displacement and repetition, two primary mechanisms, we would learn, behind hysterical symptoms, dreams, and transference. But this same persistent doubling, first brought to their attention by Anna O., is also characteristic of mimetic play which, if understood as such, admits of endless interpretations – all correct, all wrong – when seen themselves as a form of play. More importantly, this persistent doubling – as a kind of play – is especially characterized, both in her life and after her death, by the continuous emergence of two sharply delineated personae by which she came to be known.

It is widely held that Breuer was quickly engaged in extraordinary empathy with Anna O. as a result of who and what she represented from his past. Note that this beginning empathy itself is established through the conceptual experience of doubling by which Breuer's mother = Anna O.:

> It is likely that Breuer was personally driven to help [Anna O.] because she aroused the long-dormant feelings associated with his mother's death. Both of these women had the same name and, at the time she was first seen for treatment, [Anna O.] was almost exactly the age his mother had been when she died. In addition, her breakdown was precipitated by the impending death of a parent, and her illness was replete with thoughts of death. Breuer's encounter with this second, young [Anna] probably reverberated with memories of the death of his mother when he was two years old.
>
> Breger (2000, 103)

Reciprocally, the impending loss of Anna O.'s beloved father cast Breuer as an easy, convenient, and attentive paternal surrogate which was not lost on

Breuer. This much is evident from Breuer's case notes which are far more extensive than was typical of this type of report at the time. [The following details of Anna O.'s treatment are from the case notes of Dr. Josef Breuer written in 1882 at the conclusion of his treatment of her when he placed her in the "Bellevue" Sanatorium for more intensive, continued care – published in Hirschmuller (1978, 276–290)].

> [Anna O. led a] very monotonous life, limited entirely to the family; she seeks compensation in passionate fondness for her father who spoils her, and by reveling in her highly developed gifts of poetry and fantasy. Whilst everyone believed that she was paying attention she was really living out fairy tales; however, she always responded immediately when addressed so no one ever knew of this. Known as her 'private theater', this was a permanent factor in her mental life; it was all the more important – and dangerous – insofar as her excessively regimented lessons offered no outlet for natural vitality, and a wholly uneventful life gave no real content to her intellectual activities ... The sexual element is astonishingly undeveloped; I have never once found it represented even among her numerous hallucinations. At all events, she has never been in love to the extent that this has replaced her relationship with her father.
>
> 277–288

Breuer describes the original event that initiated Anna O.'s condition as she related it to him. Note Breuer's observation of the first dynamic appearance of an alternate, second state of consciousness referred to as an "absence":

> She was alone with her somnolent [drowsy, semi-conscious] father and her own anxiety, which seemed already to have been pathological. She sat on the bed, her right arm over the back of the chair, and gradually fell into a state of absence. In the course of the absence she hallucinated black snakes crawling out of the walls, and one which crawled up to her father to kill him. Her right arm had become anaesthetized owing to its position, and her fingers were transformed into small snakes with death heads (nails).
>
> 278

Breuer then reports that, as the treatment proceeded, the "absences" followed by amnesia increased. Anna O. would eventually articulate her own strange experiences in English instead of her native German:

> The absences ("time-missing" in English) giving rise to some sort of hallucination gradually multiplied; she was awake, but was not conscious

of them, though they returned more and more frequently ... When she listened, tense with anxiety, she again became quite deaf ... There have been many occasions since then when she has failed to recognize people and to understand them ... Everything we are familiar with as regards hysterical visual delusions was represented here. Seeing a death's head in place of her father; seeing a skeleton instead of him.

279

Parallel to Anna O.'s inventive means of self-expression, Breuer proceeds to construct a case "story" with an initial diagnosis based on the "strange behavior" consisting of two "extreme" states:

It was a clear case of tussis hysterica; however I classified the patient immediately as mentally ill on account of her strange behavior ... The more careful examination which now follows shows the patient's mental state to be severely disordered. Very rapid changes of mood from one extreme to another, cheerfulness, though only fairly transitory, otherwise a feeling of anxiety, pining after her father, stubborn opposition to all ... In bouts of agitation which she describes as extreme naughtiness, she throws cushions around.

280–281

According to Breuer, the two states eventually become the "two selves." Between her states of high agitation, Anna O. lucidly reports (and enacts) for Breuer her two states of consciousness:

She complains of the deep darkness in her head, how she cannot think, grows blind and deaf, has two selves, her real one and an evil one which compel her to behave badly, and so on. It became more and more evident, as we have just said, that she had two quite separate states of consciousness which tended to differ more sharply the longer the illness lasted. In one of the states she recognized her surroundings, was depressed and bad tempered but relatively normal, whilst the other produced hallucinations and she was "rude"; if at the end of this phase anything in the room had been changed, anyone entered or left, she complained that the time was lost to her, and commented on the lacuna in her conscious experience.

281

Breuer, quickly captivated, began spending several hours each day with Anna O., including both morning and evening visits. His rapt attention established, Anna O., through the guise of a second self, extended her metaphoric, somatic storytelling into literal storytelling; Breuer, and later Freud will coopt this narrative style of relating as the basis of psychoanalytic technique. Ellenburger (1970) has commented on how Anna O., in a manner uncharacteristic of her time, appeared to be leading her own treatment. Breuer describes,

> It had been observed that in her daily absences she moved within a definite phantasy world (except insofar as they produced fearful hallucinations). In the afternoon she lay in a somnolent state, and in the evenings she moaned, 'Agony, agony.' At first by chance and later – as they learned to pick up the process – by design, the others managed to pick up a word or two connected with her phantasies, and as soon as she had 'crossed over' she began to recount a story in the manner of Anderson's Picture-book or a fairy tale, first of all in her aphasic jargon [lost or altered ability to understand or express through speech], by and by as her story progressed with more polished and correct speech, until by the end of her narrative she was speaking perfectly correctly. Shortly after finishing she awoke, distinctly reassured, or – as she put it – 'gehaglich' (comfortable). During the following night she became increasingly restless, and in the morning, after two hours' sleep, she was clearly once more in another phantasy world. It was noticed, for instance, that in the daytime she would occasionally utter words such as Sandwuste (sandy desert); so when in the evening I gave her the word 'Wuste' (desert) as a cue she began to tell a story about people who had lost their way in the desert, and so on. The stories were all tragic, some very charming; most turned on the theme of a girl anxiously sitting by the side of a sick person ... If an evening passed without my hearing her story she missed the comfort which came to her on other evenings, and on the following evening she had two stories to recount.
>
> 282–283

Breuer's tentative diagnosis of hysteria is then affirmed on the basis of the intermittent, alternating appearance of symptoms with a new twist: the absences were now further articulated as "clouds," and the evening sessions were only in English, in contrast with her usual German speech during the day. Her two selves now had two languages:

> The fact that her increased psychic activity during these absences was accompanied by temporary disappearance of aphasia, together with the whole situation, led me to record a diagnosis of hysteria. I have described this matter at great length because the absences which began at sunset (which the patient later referred to as clouds (in English)), and the release and relief occasioned by telling the stories which acted as a psychic stimulus (later by reporting her hallucinations and such

like), all remained unchanged during the entire course of the illness at every stage.

283

Anna O.'s split (aphasic) language issues endured:

It is clear that exchanging one's own language for a foreign one (or making the effort to do so) was accepted by the culture of the time as a legitimate sign of illness. Anna O. was doing no more nor less than all the people she had ever heard of.

Shorter (1997, 32)

She spoke in English, but apparently without being aware of it ... We still spoke to her in German; only in moments of great anxiety was she unable to speak at all, or only in a confusion of different languages. Following the relief of her storytelling under evening hypnosis she spoke in French or Italian, so that we always knew what she would remember on the following day, and what she would not. She never had any recollection whatsoever of her 'English' evening sessions.

283

... for the best part of the day she was in a state of absence ... Strange visual disorders continued to get worse, she could not recognize people; when asked the reason for this she said that she had once been able to recognize faces just like other people without having to make a deliberate effort, whilst now in such situations she has to go through very laborious "recognizing work" (in English): the nose is like this, the hair like that, therefore this is so and so. All people were like wax figures to her, bearing no relation to her.

284

After a while it became apparent that Anna O. trusted only Breuer out of all her caretakers. This attachment developed to the degree that only he could successfully feed her when she stopped eating and drinking. At this point in the treatment, the distinguished Viennese physician and author Krafft-Ebing (2011) was called in to consult on the case (presumably by Breuer). Krafft-Ebing proceeded to administer two tests to evaluate the veracity of Anna O.'s complaints. First, he stuck a needle in her "paralyzed" leg which made her shriek. Then he lit a paper on fire and blew the smoke into her visually "impaired" eyes which caused her to go into a rage. (Apparently it wasn't just Anna O.'s symptomatic complaints that Krafft-Ebing sought to debunk: according to Freud, in his letter dated April 26, 1896, to Wilhelm Fliess, following Freud's presentation of his work on the sexual etiology of hysteria to his colleagues, Krafft-Ebing quipped, "It sounds like a scientific fairy tale" – quoted in Shur 1972, 104). Despite Krafft-Ebing's challenge to the legitimacy of Anna O.'s complaints, Breuer continued as before, capturing the ensuing escalation and intensity of Anna O.'s vacillating presentations:

> We always saw in the daytime what she would have to recount in the evening because she lived through these things and to some extent acted them out ... The change in her was remarkable when she had given her account of these matters; she came out of her absence, was at ease, cheerful, set herself to work, spent all night drawing or writing, perfectly rational, went to bed at 4 o'clock – and in the morning the same process started all over again.
>
> 285

> After her father's death she began to write left-handed.
>
> 286

> I had to work hard, pleading, chatting, and especially repeating the stereotype formula: 'There once was a boy' (in English), until she suddenly 'caught on' and began to speak. She never began without first touching my hands to make sure it was really me ... she knew that the "talking cure" (in English) would rid her of all her malice and energy, and if she did not want to be good she declined it.
>
> 286

At the end of the first summer during the treatment period, Breuer left on holiday for five weeks. What he experienced when he returned would seem to clearly indicate the interpersonal basis of her symptomatic presentation – her "bad" self clearly emerged and dominated in relation to Breuer's absence:

> I found her quite wretched, unmanageable, ill-tempered, malicious and lazy. It was apparent from her evening story telling that her resources of poetic fantasy were clearly drying up ... 'talking cures' (in English) or 'chimney sweeping' (in English) were again resorted to ... Inhibitions or acts of will (drinking, or closing her eyes to suppress tears) which occur due to affects getting stuck, as it were, until narrated away. After sunset 'cloud' (in English) hypnosis, amnesiac on awakening, in the morning no recollection of the evening ... when she narrated the phantasy the inhibition was discarded.
>
> 287–289

This passage indicates the point where Breuer, focused on an amelioration of Anna O.'s apparently distressing symptoms, began to explicitly construct an interpretation/explanation around the notion of catharsis.

[Anna O.'s most remarkable, and unexplained, symptom was not recorded in these preceding original case notes but was included by Breuer in his rewrite of the case 13 years later for publication in *Studies on Hysteria* (1957, 21–47) which he coauthored with Freud. Notes from the latter text follow]:

Breuer reported the stable continuation of the two states toward the end of the first year of treatment:

> The persisting somnambulism [sleepwalking, unconscious night activity] did not return. But on the other hand the alteration between two states of consciousness persisted. She used to hallucinate in the middle of conversation, run off, start climbing up a tree, etc. If one caught hold of her, she would very quickly take up her interrupted sentence without knowing anything about what had happened in the interval. All these hallucinations, however, came up and were reported in her hypnosis.
>
> 31

And with the development and expansion of her alternating behaviors, Breuer continued to develop and expand, in response, what he identified as the cathartic method: "I was hoping for a continuous and increasing improvement, provided that the permanent burdening of her mind with fresh stimuli could be prevented by her giving regular verbal expression to them" (32). During the final period of her treatment by Breuer Anna O. developed a remarkable symptom of "double-consciousness." Sulloway (1992) provides a popular summation of the unusual treatment events that are thought to have solidified the establishment of the cathartic cure:

> at the height of her illness, the patient regularly hallucinated the various events in her life that had actually taken place 365 days earlier ... Gradually the patient, to whom Breuer began to devote several hours each day, evolved the methodological routine of informing him, in reverse chronological order, about each and every past appearance of every symptom. She proceeded in this manner until she reached the very first moment of each symptom's appearance – at which point, to Breuer's amazement, the symptom disappeared. This was the method of 'catharsis' (Breuer's term).
>
> 55

Breuer, in his detailed description of the same period makes careful note of the *condition seconde* which continues to preoccupy him:

> A year had now passed since she had been separated from her father and had taken to her bed, and from this time on her condition became clearer and was systematized in a very clear manner. Her alternating states of consciousness, which were characterized by the fact that, from morning onwards, her *absences* (that is to say, the emergence of her

condition seconde) always became more frequent as the day advanced and took entire possession by the evening – these alternating states had differed from each other previously in that one (the first) was normal and the second alienated; now, however, they differed further in that in the first she lived, like the rest of us, in the winter of 1881-2, whereas in the second she lived in the winter of 1880-81, and had completely forgotten all the subsequent events. The one thing that nevertheless seemed to remain consistent most of the time was the fact that her father had died ... But this transfer into the past did not take place in a general or indefinite manner; she lived through the previous winter day by day. I should only have been able to *suspect* that this was happening, had it not been that every evening during the hypnosis she talked through whatever it was that that had excited her on the same day in 1881, and had it not been that a private diary kept by her mother in 1881 confirmed beyond a doubt the occurrence of the underlying events. The re-living of the previous year continued till the illness came to its final close in June 1882.

Breuer (1957, 32–33, author's emphases)

The peculiarity of the double-consciousnesses was striking though completely puzzling for Breuer who stayed in empathy with Anna O. as long as he could, reflecting an interpretive zeal that matched her modes of expression:

> Throughout the entire illness her two states of consciousness persisted side by side: the primary one in which she was quite normal psychically, and the secondary one which may well be likened to a dream in view of its wealth of imaginative products and hallucinations, its large gaps of memory and the lack of inhibition and control of its associations.

45

We finally see Breuer reach the limits of his imagination as he struggles to translate (on writing at least, and with Freud's influence) the double experience of Anna O. into the terms of his medical profession in late nineteenth-century Vienna:

> It is hard to avoid expressing the situation by saying that the patient was split into two personalities of which one was mentally normal and the other insane. The sharp division between the two states in the present patient only exhibits more clearly, in my opinion, what has given rise to a number of unexplained problems in many other hysterical patients. It was especially noticeable in Anna O. how much the products of her 'bad self', as she herself called it, affected her moral habit of mind. If these products had not been continuously disposed of, we should have been

faced by a hysteric of the malicious type – refractory, lazy, disagreeable and ill-natured; but, as it was, after the removal of those stimuli her true character, which was opposite of all these, always reappeared at once.

45–46

Breuer has finally resolved his bewilderment over the "strange behavior" of Anna O. through recourse to moralism; and concomitantly he cast his own role as one who delivers her from evil – the *condition seconde* that must be terminated. When considering the treatment in retrospect, he seems to be ambivalent, not necessarily about the technique that he developed, but regarding its conception. Breuer has noticeably stepped back from the close, if not playful, engagement with his patient. In hindsight he seemed more than wistful, almost as though he regretted being caught up in something beyond his own intentions (or chagrined at being played?):

> I have already described the astonishing fact that from beginning to end of the illness all the stimuli arising from the secondary state, together with their consequences, were permanently removed by being given verbal utterance in hypnosis, and I have only to add an assurance that this was not an invention of mine which I imposed on the patient by suggestion. It took me completely by surprise, and not until symptoms had been got rid of in this way in a whole series of instances did I develop a therapeutic technique out of it.

46

From Hirschmuller (1978) we have Anna O's own reflection on her condition written while in a sanatorium in 1882, still in the throes of the condition for which Breuer had been treating her and, importantly, immediately following his withdrawal from the case. This passage, written in non-native English, shows her measuring her condition in relation to two languages, each still associated with a different self. It also reveals her as consumed with loss – loss of her mother tongue, loss of Breuer, her father, and even "society" for the most part, along with the attention these relationships provided. (One must also take into account that she was likely addicted to morphine and chloral for sedation at this time. For at least six months post-Breuer "large amounts of chloral and morphine had been prescribed" in the sanatorium (Ellenburger 1993, 270)):

> I, a native German girl, am now totally deprived of the faculty to speak, to understand or read German. This symptom lasted during the time of a heavy nervous illness, I had to go through, in permanence longer than a year; since about 4 months it only returns regularly every evening. The physicians point it out as something strange and but rarely to be observed ... Considering my humour, my mental and psychic state during this time, there are some observations to be told. In the first

2 months of my sojourn here, I had shorter or longer absences, which I
could observe myself by a strange feeling of 'timemissing'; one told me
that I used to speak with great vivacity during these absences, but since
some weeks, there have been none. When I do not read I am laying, not
always very quiet, occupied with my thoughts, and ame quite well able
to govern them; I can reproduce the past and make plans for the future;
I only get really nervous, anxious, and disposed to cry, when the but too
well motivated fear to lose the German language for longer again, takes
possession of me. When I have society during this phase I feel much
easier, but also when I am quite alone I don't fall into heavy melancholic
or hypochondric thinking.

Hirschmuller (1978a, 296)

Over the decades following the publication of *Studies on Hysteria*, and
through various writings, Freud would undertake a retrospective historical
reinterpretation of Anna O.'s treatment. Undoubtedly, the Anna O. story
proved useful to the literary construction of his project. In nearly all of
Freud's writings he is positioning himself and the founding of psychoanalysis
as advances made on the shoulders of Breuer despite the latter's supposed
limitations. Even more importantly, the detailed clinical relationship of
Breuer and Anna O., along with its thick clinical description, would now be
incorporated into Freud's story. However, his story rested on a reconstructed
and abstracted translation of their experience:

Freud (1957, Vol. XI, all emphases from author):

> Dr Breuer's patient was a girl of twenty-one, of high intellectual gifts.
> Her illness lasted for over two years, and in the course of it she developed
> a series of physical and psychological disturbances which decidedly
> deserved to be taken seriously ... she was subject to conditions of
> *'absence'* (French term), of confusion, of delirium, and of alteration
> of her whole personality ... the enigmatic condition which, from the
> time of ancient Greek medicine, has been known as hysteria ... (10).
> [Dr. Breuer] gave her both sympathy and interest, even though, to begin
> with, he did not know how to help her. It seemed likely that she herself
> made his task easier by the admirable qualities of intellect and character
> to which he had testified in her case history.

12

Commenting on the evolution of the cathartic method, the precursor to
Freud's psychoanalytic technique of free association, Freud arrives at his
famous insight. It marks his conversion of Anna O.'s ecstatic experience
into a psychological interpretation and thus represents precisely the type
of modernist psychological storytelling that Benjamin, quoted above,
bemoaned. The further we move from the story of the actual interpersonal

clinical encounter, with its attendant surprises, strangeness, humor, pathos, concern, and overall theatricality, the more we move into a construction for which Anna O. is invoked as a useful, tragic, ancestral totem:

> Never before had anyone removed a hysterical symptom by such a method or had thus gained so deep an insight into its causation (13) ... all the pathogenic impressions came from the period during which she was nursing her sick father.
>
> 14–15

> *Our hysterical patients suffer from reminiscences.* Their symptoms are residues and mnemic symbols of particular (traumatic) experiences (16, author's emphasis) ... they remember painful experiences of the remote past, but they still cling to them emotionally; they cannot get free of the past and for its sake they neglect what is real and immediate. This fixation of mental life to pathogenic traumas is one of the most significant and practically important characteristics of neurosis.
>
> 17

> It must be emphasized that Breuer's patient, in almost all her pathogenic situations, was obliged to *suppress* a powerful emotion instead of allowing its discharge in the appropriate signs of emotion, words, or actions.
>
> 17–18

Freud goes on to explain the experience of "double-conscience" that Breuer had only described, using it to underscore his topographic dual scheme of consciousness with its division between consciousness and unconsciousness. In Freud's hands, duality becomes decidedly emblematic of conflict, not creativity:

> The study of hypnotic phenomena has accustomed us to what was at first a bewildering realization that in one and the same individual there can be several mental groupings, which can remain more or less independent of one another, which can 'know nothing' of one another and which can alternate with one another in their hold upon consciousness. Cases of this kind, too, occasionally appear simultaneously, and are then described as cases of *'double-conscience'*. If, where a splitting of the personality such as this has occurred, consciousness remains attached regularly to one of the two states, we call it the *conscious* mental state and the other, which is detached from it, the *unconscious* one.
>
> 19

Later, moving even further from the play of the original clinical experience, Freud seeks to establish his preeminence as the founder of psychoanalysis vis-à-vis Breuer in his *Autobiographical Study* (1959b). Of special note here is his story of the personal cost of displacing his elder colleague – not so much for its Oedipal connotation as for the persistent, pervasive trope of the reluctant hero who prevails at the expense of a "lesser self" or an undesirable, weaker other:

> Dr. Josef Breuer … was a man of striking intelligence and fourteen years older than myself. Our relations soon became more intimate and he became my friend and helper in my difficult circumstances. We grew accustomed to share all our scientific interests with each other. In this relationship the gain was naturally mine. The development of psychoanalysis afterwards cost me his friendship. It was not easy for me to pay such a price, but I could not escape it.
>
> 19

> The patient had recovered and had remained well and, in fact, had become capable of doing serious work. But over the final stage of the hypnotic treatment there rested a veil of obscurity, which Breuer never raised for me; and I could not understand why he had so long kept secret what seemed to me an invaluable discovery instead of making science the richer by it.
>
> 20–21

> [Breuer] might have crushed me or at least disconcerted me by pointing to his own first patient, in whose case sexual factors has ostensibly played no part whatsoever. But he never did so, and I could not understand why this was, until I came to interpret the case correctly and to reconstruct, from some remarks which he had made, the conclusion of his treatment of it. After the work of catharsis had been completed, the girl had suddenly developed a condition of 'transference love'; he had not connected this with her illness, and had therefore retired in dismay.
>
> 26

Freud (1932) reveals the details of this secretive "transference love" in a private letter to Stefan Zweig in which he further expands on the details surrounding the ending of Anna O.'s treatment. In Freud's retelling, the Anna O./Breuer story had now reached the level of tragedy. Not, as one might suppose, because Breuer "took flight" abandoning his loving patient, but because Breuer was too "conventional" and missed the opportunity to establish the hypothesized sexual longings signified by her phantom birth delivery:

> What really happened to Breuer's patient I was able to guess later on, long after the break in our relations, when I suddenly remembered something Breuer had once told me in another context before we had

begun to collaborate and which he never repeated. On the evening of the day when all her symptoms had been disposed of, he was summoned to the patient again, found her confused and writhing in abdominal cramps. Asked what was wrong with her, she replied, "Now Dr. B's child is coming!"

At this moment he held in his hand the key that would have opened the 'door to the Mothers,' but he let it drop. With all his great intellectual gifts there was nothing Faustian in his nature. Seized by conventional horror he took flight and abandoned the patient to a colleague. For months afterwards she struggled to regain her health in a sanatorium.

413

A perspective that construes events as action on an interpersonal field of mimetic play might not interpret the phantom pregnancy as the signifier of repressed sexual longings for Breuer; nor would it necessarily be interpreted as a "procreation fantasy" of a newly emerging Anna O. by virtue of her treatment (see Kimball 2000, 27). Rather, it could simply be seen as the most developed extension of the playing she had been doing from the beginning of treatment. That is, the ultimate parody of catharsis that Anna O. knew Breuer was preoccupied with – the embodied gift that she imagined he wanted and needed from her all along, an actual, other Anna O. whereby one would become two. If this was so, Breuer's uncharacteristic fear and withdrawal, his refusal to "play" and accept her gift after more than a year of sensitive and encouraging participation, would be an unexpected and intolerable rejection and loss.

Freud (1932), (reported in Forrester and Cameron 1999) writing in a private letter to his former patient Sir Arthur Tansley, continues to elaborate the tragic tale around Breuer's failure and the supposed "defect" in the treatment of Anna O. It seems he is still consumed by his singular, retrospective interpretation of her sexual repression, the uninterpreted basis of her tragic outcome:

> In Breuer's case-history, you will find a short sentence: – 'but it was a considerable time before she regained her mental balance entirely' (Studies on Hysteria, 32). Behind this is concealed the fact that, after Breuer's flight, she once again fell back into psychosis, and for a longish time – I think it was ¾ of a year – had to be put in an institution some way from Vienna. Subsequently the disease had run its course, *but it was a cure with a defect*. Today she is over 70, has never married, and, as Breuer said, which I remember well, has not had any sexual relations. On condition of the renunciation of the entire sexual function she was able to remain healthy ... It is of interest that, as long as she was active, she devoted herself to her principle concern, the struggle against white slavery.
>
> 930 (emphasis added)

Apparently, the full tragic scope of the Breuer/Anna O. treatment continues to unfold in a recently uncovered journal entry of Freud's patient, Marie Bonaparte (reported in Borch-Jacobsen 1996, 100):

> The 16th of December [1927], in Vienna. Freud told me the Breuer story. His wife tried to kill herself towards the end of Anna = Bertha's treatment. The rest is well known: Anna's relapse, her fantasy of pregnancy, Breuer's flight.
>
> Breuer to Freud: "What have you got me into?"
>
> Freud: "If you had known Breuer, he was a great mind, a mind quite superior to me. I had only one thing: courage to stand up to the majority, faith in myself ..."

It is striking to consider the extent to which Freud's ongoing narrative construction of the Anna O. story continuously correlates his seeming heroic ascendency with the tragic downfall of the other players involved. However, this makes sense in the context of what Freud himself (1959a, 149) wrote on storytelling in 1908:

> One feature above all cannot fail to strike us about the creations of these story-writers: each of them has a hero who is the center of interest, for whom the writer tries to win our sympathy by every possible means and whom he seems to place under the protection of a special Providence.

After Freud's death, psychoanalyst Ernest Jones (1953) in his epic hagiography of Freud, adopts and develops this mythic portrait of the fall of Breuer:

> Freud has related to me a fuller account than he described in his writings of the peculiar circumstances surrounding the end of this novel treatment. It seemed that Breuer had developed what we should nowadays call a strong counter-transference to his interesting patient. At all events he was so engrossed that his wife became bored at listening to no other topic, and before long jealous. She did not display this openly, but became unhappy and morose. It was a long time before Breuer, with his thoughts elsewhere, divined the meaning of her state of mind. It provoked a violent reaction in him, perhaps compounded of love and guilt, and he decided to bring the treatment to an end. He announced this to Anna O., who was by now much better, and he bade her good-by. But that evening he was fetched back to find her in a greatly agitated state, apparently as ill as ever. The patient, who according to him had appeared to be an asexual being and had never made any illusion to such a forbidden topic throughout the treatment, was now in the throes of an hysterical childbirth (pseudocyesis), the logical termination of a phantom 'pregnancy' that had been invisibly developing in response to

Breuer's ministrations. Though profoundly shocked, he managed to calm her down by hypnotizing her, and then fled the house in a cold sweat. The next day he and his wife left for Venice to spend a second honeymoon, which resulted in the conception of a daughter; the girl born in these curious circumstances was nearly sixty years later to commit suicide in New York.

224–225

Jones's dramatic account, though later soundly disputed by Hirschmuller (1978), successfully spawned a legion of (self) affirming interpretations from psychoanalysts. Blum (1998, 102) in a typical vein states "In contemporary psychoanalytic terms, [Breuer] lacked the understanding of the patient's evolving, erotic transference and his own countertransference." And Pollock (1973, 321) remarked, "In the post-termination period, her loss of Breuer probably exacerbated her initial symptoms and those of the pathological mourning which I believe were present earlier."

Over a 100 years after her treatment, Anna O. resists definitive appropriation as exhibit A for the project based on the treatment of hysteria. And so finally the efforts have stopped. Shorter (1997, 33) states,

> What did Anna O. really 'have'? In sum, she had nothing, which is to say she had what many of the other young people of her day had, namely a desire to communicate psychic distress in physical terms, and expropriate the culturally sanctioned symptoms deemed appropriate for supposedly serious illness.

Shorter goes on to assert that "it is unlikely that Anna O. ever experienced a major psychiatric illness" (25); "Indeed, the famed 'prototype of the cathartic cure' was neither a cure nor a catharsis … the illness was a creation of the mythopoetic unconscious of the patient with the unaware encouragement and collaboration of the therapist" (Ellenburger 1993, 272).

Anna O., exceptionally intelligent and creative by all accounts, wanted to play. And her play found its mimetic expression in her reflection of Breuer's intention to "cure" her; that is, cure her through this novel process they concocted together and which he deemed "catharsis." The seriousness with which Breuer undertook her treatment was matched by the earnestness with which she parodied the role of patient, always returning to self-conscious awareness, always relating to Breuer what she was up to and noting his response. As the progenitor for the psychoanalytic concept of transference, and with no aim other than mimetic play, Anna O. could remarkably analogize herself, ultimately to an embodied extent. Perhaps this accounts for her use of analogy in the only comment on psychoanalysis that she is known to have made: "Psychoanalysis in the hands of a doctor is what confession is in the hands of the Catholic priest. It depends on the user and its use whether it is a good instrument or a two-edged sword" (quoted in Edinger 1968, 15).

Freud, in the final writing of his life, perhaps betraying the basis of his long-standing allure for Anna O., wrote, "I have not been able to resist the seduction of an analogy" (Freud 1964, 268).

* * *

Annette contacted me inquiring about treatment shortly after arriving in New York City. Born and raised in Paris, France, she was attending a local university to pursue her graduate education in history. She attributed her research interest in French history to her ancestral legacy – she claimed to be a direct descendent of Duc Jean des Esseintes. As such, all areas of her life followed from what she knew of the famous aristocrat by reading Huysmans (2003). She presented as exceptionally intelligent with a wry sense of humor and exuded an attractive sophistication that seemed strangely out of synch with the fashion and interests of her peers. Her clothing, hairstyle, jewelry, style of walking and speaking, and general manner all reflected the long-lost sensibility of the late bourgeoisie, made all the more distinctive by how out of place she appeared in contemporary urban American society. Imagine a young Mrs. Havisham today. She abhorred vulgarity, profanity, and especially anything pedestrian, common, ordinary, or "standard."

Her presenting problem was an unremitting sadness, to the degree of despair, which made the execution of daily activities in her temporarily adopted home nearly impossible. It was as though her chronic sadness was the combined result of homesickness and mourning for another era along with a correlated disorientation within her current modern circumstances. So strong was her zeal for preservation and conservation that I couldn't help but wonder what dialectically other experience she was warding off, or, put differently, what modernity symbolized for her.

Georg Simmel (1964) discussed the characterological consequences of this struggle with a modern sensibility:

> The deepest problems of modern life derive from the claim of the individual to preserve the autonomy and individuality of his existence in the face of overwhelming social forces, of historical heritage, of external culture, and the technique of life.
>
> 409

its resultant "intensification of nervous stimulation" (410); and its individual human manifestation in a "blasé" and "indifferent" attitude. Simmel contrasts this with the social character of the ancient polis:

> The tremendous agitation and excitement, the unique colorfulness of Athenian life, can perhaps be understood in terms of the fact that a

people of incomparably individualized personalities struggled against the constant inner and outer pressure of a de-individualizing small town.

417–418

For lack of a better term, Simmel's student, Walter Benjamin (1996), would attribute this quality of "unique colorfulness" that permeated all levels of past societies to "porosity" (in his essay entitled "Naples" after the city where he experienced it first-hand): "Porosity results ... above all, from the passion for improvisation, which demands that space and opportunity be preserved at any price. Buildings are used as a popular stage. They are all divided into innumerable, simultaneously animated theaters" (416–417) ... "similarly dispersed, porous, and comingled is private life ... each private attitude or act is permeated by streams of communal life" (419) ... all linked through gestures "in their fastidiously specialized eroticism" (421).

Lost among the people and places far off in space and time, Annette felt at home; for in modern society, porosity had all but vanished.

> [Now] they shut themselves in houses which no-one may enter, and only there feel some measure of security ... the repugnance to being touched remains with us when we go about among people ... Even when we are standing next to them and are able to watch and examine them closely, we avoid actual contact if we can.
>
> Canetti (1993, 15)

> Perhaps the most difficult task we face daily is that of touching another person – whether the touch is physical, moral, emotional, or imaginary. Contact is crisis ... the difficulty presented by any instance of contact is that of violating a fixed boundary, transgressing a closed category where one does not belong.
>
> Carson (1990, 135)

Not only had porosity seemed to vanish, "the porousness of women," in particular, presented a threat: "sexually the female is a pore. This porous sexuality is a floodgate of social pollution ... The pores must be closed" (158–159).

I came to learn that Annette ordinarily ate very little, drank and smoked often, and was sexually quite active. Despite her ease seducing men, the liaisons rarely lasted beyond a few encounters; usually on account of her growing bored. It was really only the stimulation afforded by her immersion in her historical research that provided any sustained fulfillment. Yet once her work was complete or otherwise interrupted, she was at risk of dissolving into a mood of sadness and despair, often to an inconsolable degree. For it was then that she lived in the present, and then who was she? "Being paranoid that I might not be a person [was for her] a default condition of being a person" (Morton 2016, 31). To live this way meant that Annette trusted no one, not even herself, all seemed false to her. Yet even falseness was not without its own perverse interest for Annette:

> Often the false has a greater 'reality' than the true. Therefore, it seems that all information, and that includes anything that is visible, has its entropic side. Falseness, as an ultimate, is inextricably a part of entropy, and this falseness is devoid of moral implication.
>
> Smithson (1996a, 18)

Not surprisingly, the general theme of her historical focus was on waste and decadence, particularly as manifest in human cultural and psychological processes of entropy; a micro reflection of the macro processes by which,

> the universe would gradually run down until it reached an absolute and definitive equilibrium, without tension, just as surely as a mixture of hot and cold water gives tepid water. The end – I do not say predictable, but inevitable – would be a fall-out, or rather, not even that, a floating of dust or ashes or some kind of sickly, evenly distributed jelly, spreading out wherever its inertia might lead it.
>
> Caillois (1971, 92)

For Annette, the existential fascination with entropy implied an acute awareness of the world as "a closed system which eventually deteriorates and starts to break apart and there's no way you can really piece it back together again" (Smithson 1996b, 301).

As with most intellectual endeavors, Annette's research focus was diagnostic to the extent that it emerged in the intersection between her personal psychology and her chosen field of study (see Devereaux 1967): as such, she was the embodiment of Nietzsche's (1992) "antiquarian man":

> By tending with care to that which has existed from old, he wants to preserve for those who shall come into existence after him the conditions under which he himself came into existence – and thus he serves life. The possession of ancestral goods changes its meaning in such a soul: *they rather possess it*. The trivial, circumscribed, decaying and obsolete acquire their own dignity and inviolability through the fact that the preserving and revering soul of the antiquarian man has emigrated into them and there made its home (72–73) … When the senses of a people harden in this fashion, when the study of history serves the life of the past in such a way that it undermines continuing and especially higher life, when the historical sense no longer conserves life but mummifies it, then the tree gradually dies unnaturally from the top downwards to the

roots – and in the end the roots themselves usually perish too. Antiquarian history itself degenerates from the moment it is no longer animated and inspired by the fresh life of the present.

75 (emphasis added)

Her conservation of a bygone era in thought and action, however futile and frustrating it proved, could alternatively be viewed as a personal and political stance, as her resistance to a gnawing awareness that "every verbal exchange, every line printed, establishes communication between people, thus creating an evenness of level, where before there was an information gap and consequently a greater degree of organization" (Lévi-Strauss 1978, 413–414). The description of this process led to her high regard for Claude Lévi-Strauss, the author of *A World on the Wane* (aka *Tristes Tropiques*), in which he articulated the principles of "'entropology,' the name of the discipline concerned with the study of the highest manifestations of this process of disintegration" (414).

As interested as she was in the notion of "entropology," Annette could be vehemently dismissive of recent trends in her own discipline, especially American history. Her point of view is represented well by Aragon (1991, 35): "What is the point of remembering the names of all those presidents and admirals, oh, historians of the Starry States, if the very center of your country's ideology remains an unnamed shadowy splotch?"

Initially, I formed a tentative diagnosis of moral entropic disorder characterized by intermittent episodes of anomic lassitude as well as a chronic melancholic mood; manifest as "a kind of dotage without a fever, having for his ordinary companions fear and sadness, without any apparent occasion" (Burton 2001, I, 170). In other words, I diagnosed an endemic, multifaceted condition reflected in the constellation of her individual psychology, academic discipline, and society; "Taken together, they demonstrate the prevalence of entropy as a dominant postmodernist sentiment that expresses flatness, fragmentation, and artificiality as well as a lack of futuricity" (Gibbons 2019, 284). Given my understanding of Annette's condition as an understandable response to a larger sociocultural trend, I was determined to ignore the pathologizing prescriptions for "entropy management" in which the therapist "acts to facilitate a redirection process" (McKenzie and Murray 2013, 156).

However, it was not until I closely read Huysmans's (2003) *Against Nature* on Annette's suggestion that I began to suspect a different, more accurate etiological explanation for her suffering that even subsumed sociocultural factors. To the extent that Annette subscribed to a notion of psychological character as genetically transmitted, she completely identified with the compromised health condition of her ancestor, the Duke. He was described as a "frail young man of thirty who was anemic and highly strung, with hollow cheeks, cold eyes of steely blue, a nose which was turned up but straight and thin, papery hands" (3–4). Apparently, her genetic identification was reinforced further when she learned that "by some freak of heredity [the Duke himself] bore a striking resemblance to his distant ancestor [with] the same ambiguous expression, at once weary and wily" (4). The ensuing confusion of literary truth, historical truth, and narrative truth as an artifact of our clinical relationship would be a central issue throughout the treatment, even implicated in the current exposition.

Ordinarily,

> it is by no means to be assumed that the patient has a history (that is, a sense of historicity) at the beginning of analysis. In other words, we cannot take for granted the idea that the patient has achieved a sense of continuity of self over time, such that his past feels as if connected to his experience of himself in the present.
>
> Ogden (1989, 191)

However, in what seemed like a parodic presentation of a patient with an inversive kind of excessive historicity, Annette presented herself (consciously? unconsciously?) almost exclusively through the likenesses of the historical characters with whom she identified.

Annette confirmed this identification as she related to me that like the Duke, her emulated ancestor, in her childhood she *"would spend hours reading or daydreaming, enjoying [her] fill of solitude until night fell; and by dint of pondering the same thoughts [her] intelligence grew sharper and [her] ideas gained in maturity and precision"* (Huysmans 2003, 5) ...

> and then, reading these works, [s]he could enter into complete intellectual fellowship with the writers who had conceived them, because at the moment of conception those writers had been in a state of mind analogous to [her] own.
>
> The fact is that when the period in which a [wo]man of talent is condemned to live is dull and stupid, the artist is haunted, perhaps unknown to [her]self, by a nostalgic yearning for another age.
>
> Unable to attune [her]self, except at rare intervals, to [her] environment, and no longer finding in the examination of that environment and the creatures who endure it sufficient pleasures of observation and analysis to divert [her], [s]he is aware of the birth and development in [her]self of unusual phenomena. Vague migratory longings spring up which find fulfillment in reflection and study. Instincts, sensations, inclinations bequeathed to [her] by heredity awake, take shape and assert themselves with imperious authority. [S]he recalls memories of people and things [s]he has never known personally, and there comes a time when [s]he bursts out of the prison of her century and roams about at liberty in another period, with which, as a crowning illusion, [s]he imagines [s]he would have been more in accord.
>
> 166

As we proceeded, I remained curious as to how this antiquarian woman, this would-be Duchess, could submit to the psychotherapeutic process, itself the quintessence of modernity. Annette described her process of seeking a therapist:

> Where and when should [I] look. Into what social waters should [I] heave the lead, to discover a twin soul, a mind free of commonplace ideas, welcoming silence as a boon, ingratitude as a relief, suspicion as a haven and a harbor?
>
> 198

Following these remarks in session, I received another literarily constructed message sent from her that evening:

> You interest me. Most men are so common, so lacking in verve and poetry; but there is a depth in you, an enthusiasm and above all a serious-mindedness that warms my heart. I could become attached to you.

I now understood that all communications from Annette emanated from some source that made sense within her shifting historical and literary conception of herself. As we shall see, this was especially true of her written communications. I came to realize that recognizing the preceding quote from Sacher-Masoch (1991, 165), for example, was only half my task. A full understanding could be achieved only by grasping the intentions of each particular historical character, in this case Wanda von Dunajew or "Venus," in the context of the relationship I would be expected to reenact with her. In other words, Annette's peculiar modus operandi entering treatment involved a kind of contrived, consciously staged transference. And this would eventuate a transference-neurosis as theater (see Loewald 1980). My acceptance of this presentational trope in treatment carried serious and subtle implications.

Her knowing adoption of an historical character's voice carried the less obvious and potentially dangerous, potentially exhilarating action, of effacing Annette. This overt mimesis, this covert effacing the present with the past, or the self with another, culminated in a merging of background/foreground, subject/object and resulted in a specific (desired?) dissociative experience of depersonalization: "I know where I am, but I do not feel as though I'm at the spot where I find myself" (Caillois 1984, 30; also see Caillois 1964). People, "like insects so perfectly imitating the patterns of their [historical] habitats as to vanish completely into the uniformity of one continuous texture ... produce a continuum unimaginable for our earthly body to traverse" (Krauss 1997, 75).

Fortunately, Annette's mimetic method of historicizing herself was made somewhat sensible for me by anthropologist Michael Taussig (1993, 255):

History would seem to now allow for an appreciation of mimesis as an end in itself that takes one into the magical power of the signifier to act as if it were indeed the real, to live in a different way with the real, to live in a different way with the understanding that artifice is natural, no less than that nature is historicized. Mimetic excess as a form of human capacity potentiated by post-coloniality provides a welcome opportunity to live subjunctively as neither subject or object of history but as both, at one and the same time. Mimetic excess provides access to understanding the unbearable truths of make-believe ... namely the power to both double yet double endlessly, to become any Other and engage the image with the reality thus imagized.

Furthermore, the procedure by which the theatricality of Annette's presentation in session unfolded was meticulous and ritualized. She usually entered and sat as though posing or preparing to perform. Once cursory social amenities were dispensed with, she would take a pad from her bag onto which she had written, in French, extensive notes (a script?) from which she would then proceed to read, translating into English smoothly as she went:

> I followed a man in the street. A man of thirty or thirty-two. I wondered what you men get out of it. Oh, this time I followed at a distance. Quite good looking, backview; a sort of calm agility. It's strange how this attracts your attention. I was captivated by the whole body. When you match your step to someone else's you seem to become them in some way. He was quite different from you, this passer-by who didn't suspect a thing. I'll do it again sometime. It gave me something to think about ....

When asked, Annette was reluctant to cite her sources and grew very impatient with me. Why was I interfering with her "writing cure"? In lieu of her cooperation, I had to try and write as accurate a transcript as possible in session while she read in order to search later for her source. In this preceding passage by Aragon (1993, 167), Annette not only importantly lays out her mimetic task but she (again, consciously? unconsciously?) is suggesting to me a program for how I'm to follow her – or how we'll follow each other.

Fortunately, I had some experience with the sociological exercise of following strangers earlier in my career (Buse 2013) and was reminded of a strikingly similar passage by Baudrilliard (1988) written 60 years after Aragon's above statement. Taking the implicit direction from Annette and agreeing to play along, I found and read this passage to her:

> The other's tracks are used in such a way as to distance you from yourself. You exist only in the trace of the other, but without his being aware of it; in fact, you follow your own tracks almost without knowing it yourself ... you seduce yourself by being absent, by being no more

than a mirror for the other who is unaware ... you seduce yourself into the other's destiny, the double of his path, which, for him, has meaning, but when repeated, does not. *It's as if someone behind him knew that he was going nowhere ....*

76–77 (author's emphasis)

Over time, and as these exchanges repeated, I became aware of small, seemingly insignificant shifts in Annette's presentation each time she read to me. Her flatness of tone, her change in accent, the slowed cadence of speech, deeper breathing, and relaxed muscles around her eyes and mouth all betrayed trance behavior. By trance I refer to,

a dissociated psychological state in which individuals are noticeably disconnected from their everyday reality: they may appear to be completely withdrawn, unresponsive, see objects and people that others cannot see, and be impervious to exhaustion or to the normal passage of time.

Luhrmann (2001, 471)

Certainly, the read presentations had a performative feeling to them. Pertinent to my sessions with Annette, Yapko (2003, 65–68) and Brown and Fromm (1986, 68) have attested to the interrelationship between hypnotic trance and role-playing while Leiris (1980) describes the fundamental theatricality of trance states during possession. Bernheim (1980, 65) speaks to the hypnotic impact of a singular focus on words; a focus which seemed to enable Annette to move spontaneously into trance (Wier 1996) that was "not so much induced but evoked" through her reading (Castillo 1995, 20–21); all of which was highly conducive to the transference phenomena manifesting in our sessions (Gill and Brenman 1959, 137). Importantly, the apparent trance phenomenon was not limited to Annette; the exchanges and enactments taking place between us were mutually regressive which cast a great deal of our shared interaction in an altered, if not dissociated state (Aron and Bushra 1998).

Importantly, as observed by Bourguignon (1965), "trance states may be taken to be evidence for the occurrence of possession" (41)

... Possession, or 'mounting,' is manifested by alterations in behavior, speech, voice, facial expression, and motor behavior as well as by changes in clothing and in the manner in which the individual is responded to by others. The observer may be led to believe that a 'genuine trance' or dissociation has taken place or that some individuals may be *play acting.*

45–46 (emphasis added)

As Lewis (2003) notes, and as we will return to later, this "play acting" of possession will frequently include erotic play, sexuality and orgasm. To what extent was Annette's presentation influenced by her own historical objects of study; did *they rather possess it* as suggested earlier in Nietzsche's depiction of the antiquarian man? It all depends on how we define possession.

As we can see, regardless of its context, there does seem to be unanimity across disciplines as to the nature of possession: historian Ellenberger (1970, 13, emphasis added) states,

> An individual suddenly *seems to* lose his identity to become another person. His physiognomy changes and shows a striking resemblance to the individual of whom he is, *supposedly*, the incarnation ... In cases of lucid possession, the individual remains constantly aware of his self, but feels 'a spirit within his own spirit,' struggling against it, but cannot prevent it from speaking at times;

consider, also, this definition from the classic study of possession by Oesterreich (1966, 17, emphasis added):

> the patient's organism *appears to be* invaded by a new personality; it is governed by a strange soul ... It is *as if* another soul had entered the body and thenceforward subsisted there, in place of or side by side with the normal subject.

Finally, psychoanalyst Laing (1970, 58, emphasis added) offers,

> the individual *seems to be* the vehicle of a personality that is not his own. Someone else's personality seems to 'possess' him and to be finding expression through his words and actions, whereas the individual's own personality is temporarily 'lost' or 'gone'.

Bourguignon (1976, 10) states that "surely 'possession states' cannot exist in societies where such beliefs are absent" and in this conviction she is reinforced by Hacking's (1998) work on fugue states, in which he underscores the importance of cultural "niches" that provide the language by which we articulate psychological experience. I would suggest that determining whether Annette's trance performance, during which she appeared to be possessed, qualified as demonstrating the correct, conventional cultural and phenomenological criteria for possession is somewhat beside the point. After all, is not all classification in the human sciences ultimately based on some combination of conjecture and comparison (Ginzburg 1980)? Describing the behavioral actions in our sessions is important, as theatrical props and stage directions are important, but dwelling on the authenticity of these behavioral acts runs the risk of removing agency from the actor, Annette. Whether her trance behavior is "real" or play-acting; whether performed consciously or unconsciously; whether she was possessed or in transference (are they not phenomenologically similar?), the larger, more poignant issue for me was how these features served the over-arching mimetic character of our work. By mimetic character I am specifically referring to a *"notion of the copy, in magical practice, affecting the original to such a degree that the representation shares in or acquires the properties of the represented"* (Taussig 1993, 47, author's emphasis). This is, as Taussig notes, a disturbing notion to stay with, given its subversion of easy subject/object, and in Annette's case, past/present distinctions. (Consequently, it can seem that, "like trance before it, mimesis is in danger of becoming a reductive behaviorist explanation for possession, which would neutralize its power to disconcert" (Boddy 1994, 426). Likewise, the clinical focus on mimesis here is not to be confused with the so-called relationality of the American school of "relational" psychoanalysis (Mitchell 1988, 2000)).

Mimetic phenomena are both creative and destructive as alluded to by Caillois (2003) in his famous essay on the mimesis of insects: "Beware: Whoever pretends to be a ghost will eventually turn into one" (91). While the memetic act is creative of artifice and virtual resemblance, perhaps more importantly, it also effaces, obscures, or renders irrelevant distinctions, including the distinction between original and copy. Effacing any and all distinctions inevitably entails,

> a renunciation of the self which is analogous to the subjective evacuation which is at work in mimesis. There ... the individual makes himself disappear ... What makes mimesis so strange is precisely the fact that an organism gives up that distinction, abdicates that fundamentally vital difference between life and matter, between the organism and the inorganic.
>
> Hollier (1984, 13)

Thus, "ultimately, the mimetic drive should be regarded as an instinct of self-forgetfulness and self-loss – an instinct just as strong, if not stronger than, the instinct of self-preservation" (Hamilton 2012, 5). Unconcerned with self-preservation, and accordingly unconstrained by moral considerations, the work of mimesis lies beyond the pleasure principle. So what's to stop the work of mimesis, the dissolution of all distinctions, from being entirely subsumed by entropy tending toward generalized uniformity?

The answer is "mimetic excess," or one's own consciousness of participating as a reflection of a reflection, of the operation of mimesis itself, appearing as in a lightening flash, illuminating the derivative and contingent nature of one's being, one's environment, one's history, of nature itself. From the perspective of mimetic excess, playing along is commensurate with presenting a gift of oneself; that is, how much of myself can I expend or lose through the part I play? This is the point at which mimesis and entropy intersect with Bataille's (1991a) notions of sacrifice as a form of expenditure, and ultimately, the link between the gift, a self-incurred loss, and the renewal of the (imagined) community.

If as Caillois (2003) maintains, the world tends toward uniformity, the endpoint for the mimetic project could be a void, for mimesis would finally be irrelevant in an environment devoid of distinctions and dissymmetry, and this was precisely the environment of greatest interest for Annette. Her mimetic play, and her awareness borne of mimetic excess, spoke to her fascination, her attraction and repulsion to entropy. Yet even with my participation, the impact of her presentations required constant renewal, for their impact inevitably, continuously waned. Nor would she be satisfied repeating the same script twice. Rather, the stakes were always rising: what more of herself could she give (or lose) in order to feel distinctive, or rather, to simply feel? The most compelling, personal outlet for self-sacrifice would predictably lie in her sexuality, a foremost concern of psychotherapy, which held promise for expressing both the associative and dissociative, the creative and destructive aspects of mimesis. Bersani (1986, 20, author's emphasis) notes, "An aggressive destructiveness 'forms the basis of' human love – which, I suggest, may be another way of saying that *destructiveness is constitutive of sexuality*."

Annette's first turn toward the topic of sexuality was in the context of our discussion of her childhood and, of course, within the parameters of her discipline as well as her chosen vicarious presentation format:

> Just as Monsieur Lambercier felt for us the affection of a father, so too he had a father's authority, which he sometimes exerted to the point of inflicting common childhood punishments on us, when we had deserved this. For awhile he restricted himself to threats of punishment which were quite new to me and which I found very frightening; but after the threat had been carried out, I discovered that it was less terrible in the event then it had been in anticipation, and, what is even more bizarre, that this punishment made me even fonder of the man who had administered it. Indeed, it took all the sincerity of my affection for him and all my natural meekness to prevent me from seeking to merit a repetition of the same treatment; for I had found in the pain inflicted, and even in the shame that accompanied it, an element of sensuality which left me with more desire than fear at the prospect of experiencing it again from the same hand ... who would have believed that this ordinary form of childhood punishment, meted out to a girl of eight years by a young man of thirty, should have decided my tastes, my desires, my passions, my whole self, for the rest of my life, and in a direction that was precisely the opposite of what might naturally have been expected?
>
> Rousseau (2008, 14–15)

As per our custom, I responded by reading a passage I hoped would not only acknowledge her equation of sexual pleasure and pain but support her wish to move more deeply into it. (Despite the cool distance that writing retrospectively can provide, our exchanges at this point felt less rationally contrived and more intuitive than I am now presenting):

> Since it is true that one of man's attributes is the derivation of pleasure from the suffering of others, and that erotic pleasure is not only the negation of an agony that takes place at the same instant, but also a lubricious participation in that agony, it is time to choose between the conduct of cowards afraid of their own joyful excesses, and the conduct of those who judge that any given man need not cower like a hunted animal.
>
> Bataille (1991b, 101)

As if taking a pause (although in psychotherapy, not even pauses occur outside the narrative flow), Annette contextualized any further discussion of sexuality, particularly sadism, as she, the Duke's offspring, understood it:

> This strange and ill-defined condition cannot in fact arise in the mind of an unbeliever. It does not consist simply in riotous indulgence of the flesh, stimulated by bloody acts of cruelty ... it consists first and foremost in a sacrilegious manifestation, in a moral rebellion, in a spiritual debauch, in a wholly idealistic, wholly Christian aberration ... The truth of the matter is that if it did not involve sacrilege, sadism would have no raison d'etre ... The strength of sadism then, the attraction it offers, lies entirely in the forbidden pleasure of transferring to Satan the homage and the prayers that should go to God ... In point of fact, this vice to which the Marquis de Sade had given his name was as old as the Church itself; the eighteenth century, when it was particularly rife, had simply revived, by an ordinary atavistic process, the impious practices of the witches' sabbath of medieval times ... The same outpouring of foul-mouthed jests and degrading insults was to be seen in the works of the Marquis de Sade, who spiced his frightful sensualities with sacrilegious profanities.
>
> Huysmans (2003, 148–149)

I showed my appreciation for her linking the historical, political, and religious contexts of sexual life, beyond a solely psychological approach, and affirmed her interest in the Marquis de Sade by quoting a passage from a letter Sade wrote to his wife:

> I respect tastes, fantasies. However baroque they may be. I find them all respectable, both because one is not their master and because the most unusual and bizarre of all, if well analyzed, can always be traced back to a principle of delicacy. I shall be glad to prove this whenever you like; you know that no one else analyzes things as I do.
>
> Sade (1783, quoted in Lever 1993, 318)

With little further encouragement needed, Annette accepted the invitation and responded next session with an opening foray into the unabashed world of Sadean sexuality:

> The weather was extremely cold at the time, my little nose was running as children's usually do in the winter; I drew out a handkerchief.
>
> 'What's this/ What's this/ Be careful there,' he warned, 'I'm the one who'll attend to that operation, my sweet.'
>
> And having stretched me out upon his bed with my head a little to one side, he sat down next to me and raised my head upon his lap. He peered avidly at me, his eyes seemed ready to devour the secretion coming from my nose. 'Oh, the pretty little snotface,' said he, beginning to pant, 'how I'm going to suck her.' Therewith bending down over me, and taking my nose in his mouth, not only did he devour all the mucus between my nose and mouth, but he even lewdly darted the tip of his tongue into each of my nostrils, one after the other, and with such cleverness he provoked two or three sneezes which redoubled the flow he desired and was consuming so hungrily. But ask me for no details bearing upon this fellow, nothing appeared, and whether because he did nothing, or because he did it all in his drawers, there was nothing to be seen, and amidst the multitude of his kisses and lecherous lickings there was nothing outstanding which might have denoted an ecstasy, and consequently it is my opinion that he did not discharge. All my clothes were in place, even his hands stayed still, and I give you my word that this old libertine's fantasy might be performed upon the world's most respectable and least initiated girl without her being able to suppose there was anything lewd in it at all.
>
> Sade (1966, 276–277)

It was difficult, between sessions, on rational reflection from the perspective of today's contemporary social mores, not to be morally swayed and concerned with accusations of misogyny that so easily infiltrate a clinical relationship with an inherent imbalance of power. These concerns were somewhat assuaged for me by the research on pornography by historian Lynn Hunt. Her analysis helped me stay with the therapeutic task at hand in my current focus with Annette:

> Sade's heroines have no use for Rousseauist notions of womanhood and modesty, nor for any other strictures on woman's free disposition of her own body. Marriage, and motherhood they revile; prostitution, libertinage and abortion they consider natural rights. In a materialist universe, the only reward is bodily pleasure, and women are as entitled to that reward as any other human.
>
> Hunt (1996, 249)

Overcoming my own reticence, I offered this response to Annette:

> The whole business of eroticism is to strike to the inmost core of the living being, so that the heart stands still. The transition from the normal state to that of erotic desire presupposes a partial dissolution of the person as [s]he exists in the realm of discontinuity. Dissolution, this expression corresponds with *dissolute life*, the familiar phrase linked with erotic activity ... The whole business of eroticism is to destroy the self-contained character of the participants as they are in their normal lives.
>
> Bataille (1986, 17, author's emphasis)

In response, Annette advanced her exploration of Sade's world with increasingly explicit, graphic sexual descriptions:

> Another individual, with approximately the same tastes took me to the Tileries some few months later. He wanted me to accost men and jerk them off six inches from his face while he hid under a pile of folding chairs; and after I had jerked off seven or eight passers-by, he settled himself upon a bench by one of the most frequented of the paths, lifted my skirts from behind, and displayed my ass to all and sundry, put his prick in the air and ordered me to jerk it off well within view of half of Paris, the which, although it was at night, created such a scandal that by the time he most cynically unleashed his fuck, more than ten people had gathered around us, and we were obliged to dash away to avoid being publicly covered with shame. 'A1.'
>
> Sade (1966, 319)

Despite, or maybe due to, the increasingly explicit descriptions Annette presented, I was stuck on the simple little suffix, 'A1,' that seemed to be almost tagged on as an afterthought. I asked her about this, and she cryptically responded, *"We need the world to be organized because our reality follows from organization"* (Morin 1989, 87, emphasis added). "So, organization ratifies an experience as real?" asked I. Annette revealed, laughingly, that A was for Annette and the numbers indicated the quantity of orgasms she achieved onanistically while researching and writing the passage at home. After all, she said, when it comes to Sade, "the aim of his strategies was to induce erection and orgasm" (Beauvoir 1966, 22). I understood Annette: almost as important as the denouement in orgasm was the act of measurement leading up to it. Otherwise, how do we make play seem like more than play. Sade would concur,

> In Marseilles, [Sade] had himself whipped, but every couple of minutes he would dash to the mantelpiece and, with a knife, would inscribe on

the chimney flue the number of lashes he had just received'. His own stories were full of measurements ... [which] permits him to talk about his own delirium as if it were an external object. The process is slowed down by this excursion but his satisfaction in it is increased. The climax has to be postponed, of course, but only for a time, and the transferred fearlessness of consciousness has added to pleasure a sense of lasting possession – the illusion of everlasting possession in fact.

Bataille (1986, 194)

Annette turned to Sade's heroine Juliette, a kindred spirit, believing that "her enthusiasm for systems, organization and self-control conceal her intuition for entropy, for the restitution of a primal chaos" (Carter 1979, 103). She would no longer quote from Sade's 120 Days of Sodom, the work that "lays the foundations for a theory of perversions and prepares the metaphysics developed especially in *Juliette*" (Klossowski 1991, 73, author's emphasis). Now would come a significant step forward for her given the latter novel's different portrayal of the Sadean woman. "Juliette as narrator of her own story is responding to her own desire ... Juliette, who can proudly claim her successfully radical impropriety, can frame it into story form, is her own whore (woman)" (Gallop 1981, 62).

The life of Juliette proposes a method of profane mastery over the instruments of power. She is a woman who acts according to the precepts and also the practice of a man's world and so she does not suffer. Instead, she causes suffering.

Carter (1979, 79)

Annette read,

And the infamous one, having his wife lie full length on the couch, summons me, has me straddle her, and deposit in her open mouth the fuck that he has lately injected in my ass. Obliged to obey, I unloose a generous load and, I admit, not without a little tremor of wickedness I gaze down to see virtue thus so cruelly humiliated by vice ... And the tempo of these infamies increased apace; the infamous one promised two euros to whoever of us three most successfully teased the victim; the rules of the game admitted blows of the fist, kicks, bites, slaps, pinches, indeed, there were hardly any rules at all; and the scoundrel jerked himself off while observing the contest. 'A1.'

Sade (1968, 138–139)

It was exceedingly important that I receive Annette's presentation of Juliette as the powerful statement she intended it to be. To that end, I reflected on Juliette, whose capacity to destroy turns her into an entirely paradoxical and antinomical being, resembling the forces of nature which can equally create and destroy with benevolent grace and an indifferent cruelty, defying judgement, moving beyond the realms of innocence and guilt.

Kamperidis (2011, xiii)

Annette, presumably encouraged by my characterization, delved deeper into her emulation of Juliette (who here is emulating Clairwil):

It was not long before the ill-starred lovers were both in the most deplorable state imaginable. Not yet in a position to judge Clairwil, her cruelty, I must confess, startled me; but when I saw her turn to execrations of a very different kind, when I saw her daubing her cheeks with the victim's blood, tasting it, drinking it, when I saw her bite into his flesh and tear it away with her teeth; when I saw her rub her clitoris on the bleeding wounds she opened in the wretch, when I heard her cry, 'Juliette, come do as I am doing'; then, urged to it by this wild beast, carried away by her hideous example – ah, my friends, must I own that I imitated her? Nay, the truth may well be that I surpassed her; I may even have led the way, stimulated her imagination by atrocities which would not have occurred otherwise; perhaps, who knows? For I waxed furious too, my every nerve was afire, my very perverse soul revealed itself in its entirety; and I discovered that devouring the flesh of a man could have as powerful an effect upon my senses as lashing a woman to ribbons. 'A1', 'A2.'

Sade (1968, 364)

We had reached an extreme, the only Sadean transgression left unvisited was murder, and with that, a final extinguishing of the self. Sontag (1983, 225) states: "Death is the only end to the odyssey of the pornographic imagination when it becomes systematic, that is, when it becomes focused on the pleasures of transgression rather than mere pleasure itself." I observed our predicament in my response to Annette:

We are lost on inaccessible heights. Nothing remains that is hesitant or moderative. In an endless and relentless tornado, the objects of desire are invariably propelled toward torture and death. The only conceivable end is possible desire of the executioner to be the victim of torture himself. In Sade's will ... this instinct reached its climax by demanding that not even his tomb should survive: it led to the wish that his very name should 'vanish from the memory of men.'

Bataille (1993, 116)

It appeared that Annette had reached her limit, a limit also known to Sade; "as Bataille saw it, Sade's writing was compelled by a death wish, an impossible desire to be 'released' through self-destruction" (Dean 1994, 188). Sade, locked for years in the Bastille; Annette, isolated and dejected in the middle of New York City, each trying to write their way out. And now, after all, it seemed our historical-literary pas de deux must have finally exhausted itself.

Annette entered the next session somewhat more distant than usual making little or no eye contact. She reported having had a dream about me and asked me if I wanted to hear it. I said of course I did. In an apparently embarrassed and apologetic manner she reported that she dreamt I turned into Killer Bob (see Figure 10.2). She explained that she was referring to,

> a fictional character and the main antagonist of the television series Twin Peaks. He is an interdimensional entity who feeds on pain and sorrow. He possesses human beings and then commits acts of rape and murder in order to feast upon his victims.
>
> Wikipedia (2020)

When I asked about her reticence to tell me this dream she said that she didn't want to insult me. I did not buy this. She composed a dream in which she had me murdered and replaced by Bob. I told her that if I was now Bob, it was only to grant her, us, license to be equally wild and transgressive, that is, to sanction murder. I unequivocally accepted the transference of Bob.

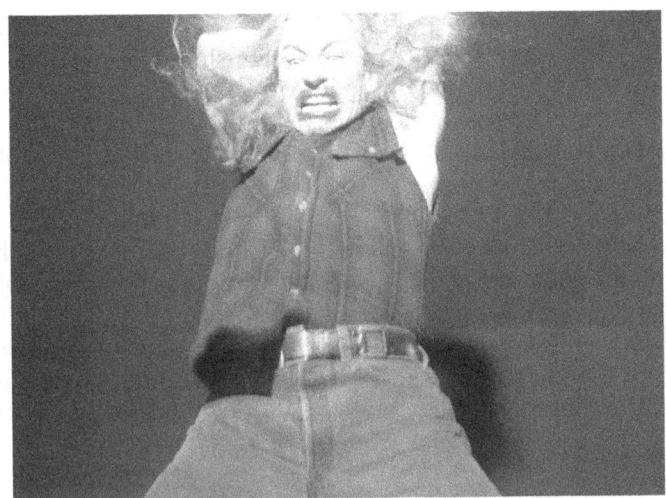

Figure 10.2 Killer Bob from the television series "Twin Peaks."
Source: Courtesy of Twin Peaks Productions, Inc. and CBS Home Entertainment, Inc.

Annette followed this session with another presentation. This time using her preselected script to address me, Bob, directly head-on as she had not done before:

> I don't especially want you only to visit low sorts of women. I imagine you with different mistresses, my dearest, and it helps me to fill up my days of seclusion. I imagine one who you say is so common, and the other, the one I give to you without knowing her: a tall brunette, a little uppity whom you must try and find. I don't pretend for a minute that she has all the advantages over me, certainly not. But it's not a gift to turn your nose up at. When I'm alone I enjoy bringing you together but I don't forget I love you and I allow myself a little jealousy. I imagine your body, your movements, her refusals then ... ah, I'm crazy. She behaves strangely in all this. My dear, in my imagination I avenge myself on your accomplice for your numerous infidelities. Please, do it for me. You see how you come into my innermost thoughts 'A1.'
>
> Aragon (1993, 165–166)

Annette could now face me while imagining her desire *en absentia*; she could release herself with the thought of me engaging with a copy of her.

In the same way that the earlier texts by Sade had less to do with sex than transgression, Annette's presentation through Aragon had less to do with sex than seduction. And seduction lent itself perfectly to her personal goal of losing herself for reasons explored by Baudrilliard (1990) which I shared with her:

> Seduction does not consist of a simple appearance, nor a pure absence, but the eclipse of the presence. Its sole strategy is to be-there/not-there, and thereby produce a sort of flickering, a hypnotic mechanism that crystallizes attention outside all concern with meaning. Absence here seduces presence ... Everything is finery in this sense, and belongs to the genius of appearance.
>
> 85–86

I immediately realized my misstep; I had exposed Annette's artifice and by identifying her seductive sleight of hand, I too was now raising the stakes of our work. Unmasking her risked the dreaded entropic slide into the ordinariness she abhorred – reduced to "a patient" with complexes to be interpreted, reducing our play to her "treatment." She returned the following session to present a script of her own composition, her first, for the last time. Again, she addressed me directly:

> I entered your office and you sneered at me saying A is not for Annette, A is for ... is for An ... Anna ... Animale ... ANIMALE! Then you told me to get on all fours on the sofa just where I'm sitting right now.

After spanking me for a while you slowly removed my pants then my underwear. You fingered me vaginally …'A1,' then you fingered me anally and vaginally simultaneously …'A2,' you didn't stop but started spanking me very hard while fingering me …'A3,' and finally, you got up astride me and pleasured yourself onto my bruised, raw pink and bloody ass …'A4.' I was too weak to move while you rubbed the pink mixture of your semen and my blood with your left hand in a counterclockwise spiral motion around my ass.

I asked what was most important to her about her story. She retorted, "You spent yourself on me, not in me."

With that the session ended and she left. I turned out the lights and sat there, my office lit only by the streetlamps outside. Nothing. After a while like this I thought I heard something at my door. I went to check and saw Annette in the bright hallway. "Wow, you scared the shit out of me," I exclaimed. Without a word she entered my dark waiting room, a silhouette, placed her hand around my neck and pulled me toward her. She kissed me on the lips, thereby terminating her treatment, turned around, and walked out.

* * *

Freud began *Studies on Hysteria* by addressing the ethical consideration of the privacy of the patients presented in its pages:

> Our experience is derived from private practice in an educated and literate social class. And the subject matter with which we deal often touches upon our patients' most intimate lives and histories. It would be a grave breach of confidence to publish material of this kind, with the risks of the patients being recognized and their acquaintances becoming informed of facts which were confided only to the physician.
>
> 1957, xxix

Despite this pledge of confidentiality for his patients, Ernest Jones, psychoanalyst and Freud's biographer, would reveal Anna O.'s true identity to the world after Freud's death. Jones (1953, 223) simply stated, "Since she was the real discoverer of the cathartic method, her name, which was actually Bertha Pappenheim, deserves to be mentioned." Of course, it all seems inevitable now. Psychoanalysts above all know that secrets secrete. Paraphrasing Foucault (1990, 35, author's emphasis): "What is peculiar to psychoanalysts, in fact, is not that they consigned Bertha Pappenheim to a shadow existence, but that they dedicated themselves to speaking about her *ad infinitum*, while exploiting her as Anna O."

Pappenheim was concerned that as few people as possible know she was 'Anna O.' After the publication of Studies on Hysteria in 1895 by Freud and Breuer, her identity as 'Anna O.' although widely known in upper-class Viennese Jewish community, was known to only a few relatives and close colleagues in Frankfurt.

Kimball (2000, 22)

Nothing at all was known to her friends and coworkers, and Jones' unauthorized disclosure came as a great shock. Bertha Pappenheim had never mentioned this period of her life and violently opposed any suggestion of psychoanalytic therapy for someone she was in charge of, to the surprise of her coworkers ... Her complete silence about her years during Breuer's and later treatment is surprising since she liked to talk about herself, her parents, her education, her trips, meetings and her collections.

Edinger (1968, 15)

"Bertha Pappenheim's surviving relatives and friends were deeply offended by Jones' disclosure" (Hirschmuller 1978, 95).

And then suddenly there were two identifiably distinct personae: Anna O. and Bertha Pappenheim. And like Anna O., Bertha Pappenheim sought a creative outlet in her storytelling; only now written, not enacted or spoken.

She was not cured until she took complete control of language and subjectivity in her own writing ... Anna O. recovered completely only with the publication of her first book, In the Rummage Shop, in 1890. Rather than continuing her role as the passive hysterical patient, through writing she became one who controlled her own cure.

Showalter (1993, 316)

In the Rummage Shop (Pappenheim 2008) is replete with tragic themes of loss, grief, and mourning. Gillman (2008), in his introduction, notes, "Story telling is the road to cure" (10) ..."when you read her writing, it remains a monument to a way of imagining life as part of an affective thought experiment, one centered in the culture of nineteenth-century Germany but able in complex ways to transcend it" (13)

... Pappenheim's writings reveal a great deal about her sense of a world in flux over which she feels empowered. When we read them, we are placed within this oddly optimistic world of literature as a tool for 'life improvement,' which the moderns dismissed as old-fashioned and unaesthetic ... she was in no ways 'modern' but very much a writer of works of self-improvement.

15–16

Kimball (2008, 30) adds to this notion of Bertha's self-help writing,

Writing was an important part of her self-reconstruction, because through it she was able to make connections between her internal worlds of fantasy and the external worlds of other people's realities, to act on the world, to make change, and to inspire others to act in accordance with her visions.

And Breger (2000, 109) concurs,

> Bertha's writing and work were major factors in her recovery. The 'private theater' of her childhood was the precursor to the literary compositions of adult years. In addition to her poetry and fairy tales, she wrote plays, a translation and a preface to Mary Wollstonecraft's *Vindication of the Rights of Women*, newspaper articles, and polemical pieces.

The following poem by Bertha, entitled "Love did not come to me" (written in 1911 and reported in Hirschmuller 1978b, 308), is representative of both her preoccupation with the tragedy of lost opportunity as well as her efforts to compensate for it. It addresses, albeit poetically, the same subject that Freud had offhandedly identified as her "defect":

> Love did not come to me –
> So I live like the plants,
> In the cellar, without light
> Love did not come to me –
> So I sound like a violin
> With a broken bow
> Love did not come to me –
> So I bury myself in work
> And, chastened, live for duty.
> Love did not come for me –
> So I like to think of death
> As a friendly face.

That writing can resemble, if not actually replicate, the benefits of the therapeutic process has been persuasively argued (see Schafer 1978; Spence 1982; Brooks 1994). Yet in spite of the widely held belief that Bertha Pappenheim was "cured" through her writing, certain aspects of Anna O.'s experience endured. Specifically, Bertha still sought to mimetically express herself through the adoption of an alternate persona. First, in the adoption of a pseudonym to publish her stories (Paul Berthold); and second, in a profound mimetic emulation of her own ancestor:

> She sought out female models, first in Mary Wollstonecraft, the pioneer of the feminist movement, and then in an ancestor, Gluckel von Hameln, who exemplified these same qualities. She had her picture painted, dressed in this woman's clothes, entitled 'Bertha Pappenheim

as Gluckel.' These identifications enabled her to construct a new self out of the fragments of her old life.

Breger (2000, 109)

Pollack (1971) elaborates on Bertha's identification with her ancestor:

> Bertha Pappenheim seemingly had the capacity for significant identifi-
> cations which could be modified or transformed ... Bertha seemingly
> utilized Gluckel as a model for her own work with young people, and as an
> identification figure that assisted in the consolidation of her feminine self.
>
> 216
>
> The translation of Gluckel's memoirs by Bertha Pappenheim is one of
> the first of her writings in which she uses her own feminine name. The
> publication of this translation may well herald the resolution of Bertha
> Pappenheim's identity conflict. Her personality became integrated
> along the feminine axis and her life became modeled after Gluckel. As
> an adult, Bertha Pappenheim is seen as a religious, selfless, devoted,
> charitable, aggressive woman, fighting for her ideals as they related to
> aid for the helpless, the weak, the disenfranchised and the oppressed.
>
> 219

[and] "she wanted to look like old Gluckel" (220).

"Not only did Bertha Pappenheim want to look like her most famous ancestress ... whose words of homely wisdom she often quoted, but that bright, energetic, deeply religious mother was clearly her ideal woman" (Edinger 1968, 18). It is a tribute to Bertha that her ancestor-identification led to a distinguished reputation as a proto-feminist, among the first in Germany, as well as Germany's first social worker with 40 years devoted to philanthropic social work (Swenson 1994). Kimball (2000, 28) notes,

> Although she never had biological children, she was involved in the lives
> of hundreds of children in her work at the orphanage [as headmistress]
> (1895–1906) and in her own institution at Isenburg (1907–1936). She
> identified closely with the ideology of spiritual motherhood that was so
> central to German maternal feminism.

So, what place did Anna O.'s pioneering psychoanalytic encounter ultimately find in Bertha Pappenheim's life? The past experience with the two doctors became the stuff of dreams; though notably still exhibiting the playful splitting among two personae. The following is one of her self-recorded dreams (in 1911, reported in Edinger 1968):

> I've got to tell you about a dream. I was dreaming that I told my mother I
> tamed two jackals. Mama would not believe me; so I brought them and,

though I was previously quite sure that these were two jackals I now saw myself that I had two cats on a leash. I got angry, I pulled the leash, and it was Mr. H and Mr. S. Mama graciously asked them to sit down in the dining room on Leerbachstrass (the home of Bertha Pappenheim while her mother was alive). Yet my stateroom actually smelled of real jackals.

40

Finally, Bertha approached her death as she lived her life – playfully. She authored the end of her story on her own terms, as someone who always understood that "all narration is obituary in that life acquires definable meaning only at, and through, death" (Brooks 1977, 284). Bertha Pappenheim's self-composed obituary (1934) appeared in Family News on her death in 1936 (as reported in Edinger 1968, 99): "She was a woman who for decades stubbornly fought for her ideas. Ideas of her times. But she did this by ways and means which tried to anticipate developments and were not to everybody's taste. What a pity!"

* * *

After some years marked only by occasional polite holiday greetings, I finally crossed paths with Annette during one of her rare visits to New York. She reported that she had returned to Paris where she was writing her dissertation. After many starts and stops she had finally commenced, with faculty approval, a historical-literary analysis of Odette de Crecy, a central character from Proust's (2003) Swann's Way. As she discussed her research with me it became clear that she, again, had developed an identification with a fictitious character. I wondered to myself if the impact of our therapeutic work could be measured by the difference between her previous identification with the Duc Jean des Esseintes and Odette.

If Annette's choice of literary identification didn't betray a meaningful change in her life, then it seemed her new lifestyle did. She reported that she was not in a relationship, lived an asexual life, and regularly followed an ascetic routine. She wrote every morning in the university library. She attended dharma lectures in the evening and explored several paths of self-improvement presented in mainstream popular publications. With the predictable zealousness of the convert, Annette was eager to share these self-affirming insights with me. Her current reading reassured her that "In practice, you can be in pain but you need not suffer" (Burch and Penman 2015, 74). I was struck by the distance she had come from the world as we once understood it, framed by the thought of Bataille, who would have held this platitude of a promise in contempt: "Pain shaped my character. In school, with my frostbitten fingers – pain is the teacher. 'Without your pain, you're nothing!'" (Bataille 1988, 69); or,

Anyone who, slyly, wants to avoid suffering confuses himself with the entirety of the universe, judges each thing as if he were it, in the same way that he imagines, at bottom, he will never die. We receive these hazy illusions with life like a narcotic necessary to bear it. But what happens to us when, disintoxicated, we learn what we are?

Bataille (2014, 4)

Asked if she did not feel lonely, she framed her solitude as a choice, a pragmatic means to an end. She believed that one way to inure herself to metropolitan life was to detach from others, if not bodily than at least cognitively. She was supported in this view by another favored reading, "The Practice of Intentional Solitude": "Truly the only thing one needs for intentional solitude is the ability to tune out distractions. A woman can learn to detach from other people, noise, and chatter" (Estes 1997, 317–318). Evidently, her reading was selected to rationalize her isolation. To wit, from yet another favorite: "When you have made good friends with yourself, your situation will be more friendly too" (Chodron 2005, 8).

These truisms, platitudes, and the overall solipsism struck me as defensive, as an impregnable wall around her, perhaps even a (necessary?) repudiation of our work together. Was it as Modell (1975) argued: that a fear of the perceived intrusiveness of the other and an aversion to outside influence had led to an illusory sense of self-sufficiency and autonomy? Or was this simply the entropic process that so beguiled Annette finally manifesting in a calm, albeit disquieting personal stasis?

I searched her eyes for any sign of the playful abandon that once defined her, and us, but it was gone.

And so, in an attempt to revitalize Annette's amorous and unvarying attitude toward me, to which I was afraid of responding, I decided I would write about her, finally, in an essay posing a disguised but sincere challenge of her wish to take care ....

Proust (2003, 319)

Now what's going to happen to us without barbarians?
They were, those people, a kind of solution.

Cavafy (1898)

Bibliography

Aragon, Louis. *Treatise on Style*. Translated by Alyson Waters. Lincoln, NE: University of Nebraska Press, 1991/1928.

Aragon, Louis. "The French Woman." In *The Libertine*, 161–185. Edited by Louis Aragon. Translated by Jo Levy. New York: Riverrun Press, 1993/1924.

Aron, Lewis and Annabella Bashra. "Mutual Regression: Altered States in the Psychoanalytic Situation." In *Journal of the American Psychoanalytic Association*, 389–412. Vol. 46, 1998.

238 The end(s) of psychotherapy

Bataille, Georges. *Erotism: Death and Sensuality.* San Francisco, CA: City Lights Books, 1986/1957.

Bataille, Georges. *Guilty.* Translated by Bruce Boone. Venice, CA: Lapis Press, 1988/1961.

Bataille, Georges. "The Notion of Expenditure." In *Visions of Excess: Selected Writings, 1927–1939,* 116–129. Edited and translated by Allan Stoekl. Minneapolis, MN: University of Minnesota Press, 1991a/1933.

Bataille, Georges. "The Use Value of D. A. F. de Sade (An Open Letter to my Current Comrades)." In *Visions of Excess: Selected Writings, 1927–1939,* 91–102. Edited and translated by Allan Stoekl. Minneapolis, MN: University of Minnesota Press, 1991b/1930.

Bataille, Georges. "Solar Anus." In *Visions of Excess: Selected Writings, 1927–1939,* 5–9. Edited and translated by Allan Stoekl. Minneapolis, MN: University of Minnesota Press, 1991c/1931.

Bataille, Georges. *Literature and Evil.* New York: Marion Boyars, 1993.

Bataille, Georges. *Inner Experience.* Translated by Stuart Kendall. Albany, NY: State University of New York Press, 2014/1954.

Baudrilliard, Jean. "Please Follow Me." In *Suite Venitienne,* 75–86. Translated by Dany Barash and Danny Hatfield. Seattle, WA: Bay Press, 1988.

Baudrilliard, Jean. *Seduction.* Translated by Brian Singer. New York: St. Martin's Press, 1990/1979.

Beauvoir, Simone de. "Must We Burn Sade?" In *The 120 Days of Sodom and Other Writings,* 3–64. Compiled and translated by Austryn Wainhouse and Richard Seaver. New York: Grove Press, 1966/1955.

Benjamin, Walter. "Naples." In *Walter Benjamin: Selected Writings, Volume 1, 1913–1926,* 414–421. Edited by Marcus Bullock and Michael W. Jennings. Translated by Edmund Jephcott. Cambridge, MA: Belknap Press, 1996/1925.

Benjamin, Walter. "The Storyteller: Observations on the Works of Nikolai Leskov." In *Walter Benjamin: Selected Writings, Volume 3, 1935–1938,* 143–166. Edited by Howard Eiland and Michael W. Jennings. Translated by Edmund Jephcott. Cambridge, MA: Belknap Press, 2002/1936.

Bernheim, Hippolyte. *Bernheim's New Studies in Hypnotism.* Translated by Richard S. Sandor. New York: International Universities Press, 1980/1891.

Bersani, Leo. *The Freudian Body: Psychoanalysis and Art.* New York: Columbia University Press, 1986.

Blum, Harold P. "From Suggestion to Insight, from Hypnosis to Psychoanalysis." In *Freud: Conflict and Culture,* 94–104. Edited by Michael S. Roth. New York: Alfred A. Knopf, 1998.

Boddy, Janice. "Spirit Possession Revisited: Beyond Instrumentality." In *Annual Review of Anthropology,* 407–434. Vol. 23, 1994.

Borch-Jacobsen, Mikkel. *The Emotional Tie: Psychoanalysis, Mimesis, and Affect.* Stanford, CA: Stanford University Press, 1993.

Borch-Jacobsen, Mikkel. *Remembering Anna O.: A Century of Mystification.* Translated by Kirby Olson. New York: Routledge, 1996.

Botting, Fred and Scott Wilson. "Literature as Heterological Practice: Georges Bataille, Writing and Inner Experience." In *Textual Practice,* 195–207. Vol. 7 (2), 1993.

Bourguignon, Erika. "The Self, the Behavioral Environment, and the Theory of Spirit Possession." In *Context and Meaning in Cultural Anthropology,* 39–60. Edited by Melford Spiro. New York: Free Press, 1965.

Bourguignon, Erika. *Possession*. Prospect Heights, IL: Waveland Press, 1976.

Breger, Louis. *Freud: Darkness in the Midst of Vision*. New York: John Wiley & Sons, 2000.

Breuer, Josef. "The Case History of Bertha Pappenheim (Anna O.)." In *The Life and Work of Josef Breuer: Physiology and Psychoanalysis*, 276–290. Edited by Albrecht Hirschmuller. New York: New York University Press, 1978/1882.

Breuer, Josef and Sigmund Freud. "Studies on Hysteria." In *The Standard Edition of the Complete Psychological Works of Sigmund Freud, Volume II*, ix–335. Edited and translated by James Strachey. London: Hogarth Press, 1957/1895.

Brooks, Peter. "Freud's Masterplot: Questions of Narrative." In *Literature and Psychoanalysis, The Question of Reading: Otherwise*, 280–300. New Haven, CT: Yale French Studies. Vols 55/56, 1977.

Brooks, Peter. *Psychoanalysis and Storytelling*. Cambridge, MA: Blackwell, 1994.

Brown, Daniel P. and Erika Fromm. *Hypnotherapy and Hypnoanalysis*. Hillsdale, NJ: Lawrence Erlbaum Associates, 1986.

Burch, Vidyamala and Danny Penman. *You are Not Your Pain: Using Mindfulness to Relieve Pain, Reduce Stress, and Restore Well-being*. New York: Flatiron Books, 2015.

Burton, Robert. *The Anatomy of Melancholy*. New York: New York Review of Books Publishing, 2001/1621.

Buse, William. "Through the Looking Glass and Back Again: The Following Exercise." In *Anthropology & Humanism*, 107–121. Vol. 38 (2), 2013.

Caillois, Roger. *The Mask of Medusa*. Translated by George Ordish. New York: Clarkson N. Potter, 1964.

Caillois, Roger. "Dynamics of Dissymmetry." In *Diogenes*, 62–92. Translated by Mary Fradier. Vol. 76, 1971.

Caillois, Roger. "Mimesis and Legendary Psychasthenia." Translated by John Shepley. In *October*, 17–32. Vol. 31, 1984/1935.

Caillois, Roger. *Man, Play, and Games*. Translated by Meyer Barash. Chicago, IL: University of Illinois Press, 2001/1958.

Caillois, Roger. "Mimesis and Legendary Psychasthenia." In *The Edge of Surrealism: A Roger Caillois Reader*, 89–103. Edited by Claudine Frank. Translated by Claudine Frank and Camille Naish. Durham, NC: Duke University Press, 2003/1935.

Canetti, Elias. *Crowds and Power*. Translated by Carol Stewart. New York: Farrar, Straus, and Giroux, 1993.

Carson, Anne. "Putting Her in Her Place: Woman, Dirt, and Desire." In *Before Sexuality: The Construction of Erotic Experience in the Ancient Greek World*, 135–169. Edited by David M. Halperin, John J. Winkler, and Froma I. Zeitlin. Princeton, NJ: Princeton University Press, 1990.

Carson, Anne. "The Gender of Sound: Description, Definition, and Mistrust of the Female Voice in Western Culture." In *Resources for Feminist Research/DRF*, 24–30. Vol. 23 (3), 1994.

Carter, Angela. *The Sadeian Woman and the Ideology of Pornography*. New York: Pantheon Books, 1979.

Castillo, Richard J. "Culture, Trance, and the Mind-brain." In *Anthropology of Consciousness*, 17–34. Vol. 6 (1), 1995.

Cavafy, Constantine P. "Waiting for the Barbarians." Edited and translated by Edmund Keeley and Philip Sherrard. In *Voices of Modern Greece*, 7–8. Princeton, NJ: Princeton University Press, 1981/1898.

Chodron, Pema. *When Things Fall Apart*. Boston, MA: Shambhala, 2005.

Cixous, Helene and Catherine Clement. *The Newly Born Woman*. Translated by Betsy Wing. Minneapolis, MN: University of Minnesota Press, 1986.

Dean, Carolyn. *The Self and Its Pleasures: Bataille, Lacan, and the History of the Decentered Subject*. Ithaca, NY: Cornell University Press, 1994.

Devereaux, Georges. *From Anxiety to Method in the Social Sciences*. The Hague: Mouton & Co., 1967.

de Sade, Marquis. *The 120 Days of Sodom and Other Writings*. Compiled and translated by Austryn Wainhouse and Richard Seaver. New York: Grove Weidenfeld Press, 1966/1785.

de Sade, Marquis. *Juliette*. Translated by Austryn Wainhouse. New York: Grove Press, 1968/1797.

de Sade, Marquis. "Letter to Madame Sade." In *Sade: A Biography*, 318. Written and edited by Maurice Lever. Translated by Arthur Goldhammer. New York: Harcourt, Brace & Company, 1993/1783.

Edinger, Dora. *Bertha Pappenheim: Freud's Anna O.* Highland Park, IL: Congregation Solel, 1968.

Ellenberger, Henri F. *The Discovery of the Unconscious: The History and Evolution of Dynamic Psychiatry*. New York: Basic Books, 1970.

Ellenberger, Henri. *Beyond the Unconscious: Essays of Henri F. Ellenberger in the History of Psychiatry*. Edited by Mark S. Micale. Translated by Françoise Dubor and Mark S. Micale. Princeton, NJ: Princeton University Press, 1993.

Estes, Clarissa Pinkola. *Women Who Run with the Wolves: Myths and Stories of the Wild Woman Archetype*. New York: Ballantine Books, 1997.

Forrester, John. "The True Story of Anna O." In *The Seductions of Psychoanalysis: Freud, Lacan, and Derrida*, 17–29. Edited by John Forrester. New York: Cambridge University Press, 1994.

Forrester, John and Laura Cameron. "'A Cure with a Defect': A Previously Unpublished Letter by Freud Concerning 'Anna O.'." In *International Journal of Psychoanalysis*, 929–942. Vol. 80, 1999.

Foucault, Nichel. *The History of Sexuality, Volume 1: An Introduction*. Translated by Robert Hurley. New York: Vintage Books, 1990.

Freeman, Lucy. *The Story of Anna O*. New York: Walker and Company, 1972.

Freud, Sigmund. "Five Lectures on Psychoanalysis." In *The Standard Edition of the Complete Psychological Works of Sigmund Freud, Volume XI*, 3–56. Edited and translated by James Strachey. London: Hogarth Press, 1957/1909.

Freud, Sigmund. "Creative Writers and Day-dreaming." In *The Standard Edition of the Complete Psychological Works of Sigmund Freud, Volume IX*, 141–154. Edited and translated by James Strachey. London: Hogarth Press, 1959a/1908.

Freud, Sigmund. "An Autobiographical Study." In *The Standard Edition of the Complete Psychological Works of Sigmund Freud, Volume XX*, 3–74. Edited and translated by James Strachey. London: Hogarth Press, 1959b/1925.

Freud, Sigmund. "Constructions in Analysis." In *The Standard Edition of the Complete Psychological Works of Sigmund Freud, Volume XXIII*, 255–269. Edited and translated by James Strachey. London: Hogarth Press, 1964/1937.

Freud, Sigmund. "Letter to Stefan Zweig." In *The Letters of Sigmund Freud*, 412–413. Edited by Ernst L. Freud. Translated by Tania and James Stern. New York: Basic Books, 1975/1932.

Gallop, Jane. Intersections: *A Reading of Sade with Bataille, Blanchot, and Klossowski*. Lincoln, NE: University of Nebraska Press, 1981.

Gibbons, Alison. "Entropology and the End of Nature in Lance Olsen's *Theories of Forgetting*." In *Textual Practice*, 280–299. Vol. 33 (2), 2019.

Gill, Merton M. and Margaret Brenman. *Hypnosis and Related States: Psychoanalytic Studies in Regression*. New York: John Wiley & Sons, 1959.

Gillman, Sandor. "Introduction." In *In the Junk Shop and Other Stories*, 7–20. Edited by Berthe Pappenheim. Riverside, CA: Ariadne Publishing, 2008.

Ginzburg, Carlo. "Morelli, Freud and Sherlock Holmes: Clues and Scientific Method." Translated by Anna Davin. In *History Workshop*, 5–36. Vol. 9, Spring, 1980.

Guttmann, Melinda G. *The Enigma of Anna O.: A Biography of Bertha Pappenheim*. Wickford, RI: Moyer Bell, 2001.

Hacking, Ian. *Mad Travelers: Reflections on the Reality of Transient Mental Illnesses*. Charlottesville, VA: University Press of Virginia, 1998.

Hamilton, John. "The Luxury of Self-destruction: Flirting with Mimesis with Roger Caillois." Presented at *Flirtations: Rhetoric and Aesthetics This Side of Seduction, a Poetics and Theory/Comparative Literature Workshop*, Draper Program, New York University, March 3, 2012. Retrieved from dash.harvard.edu.

Hirschmuller, Albrecht. *The Life and Work of Josef Breuer: Physiology and Psychoanalysis*. New York: New York University Press, 1978.

Hollier, Denis 1984. "Mimesis and Castration 1937." Translated by William Rodarmor. In *October*, 3–15. Vol. 31 Winter, 1984.

Huizinga, Johan. *Homo Ludens: A Study of the Play-element in Culture*. Boston, MA: Beacon Press, 1955.

Hunt, Lynn. *The Invention of Pornography: Obscenity and the Origins of Modernity, 1500–1800*. New Yok: Zone Books, 1996.

Hunter, Dianne. "Hysteria, Psychoanalysis, and Feminism: The Case of Anna O." In *Feminist Studies*, 464–488. Vol. 9 (3), 1983.

Huysmans, Joris-Karl. *Against Nature (A Rebours)*. Translated by Robert Baldick. New York: Penguin Books, 2003/1884.

Jones, Ernest. *The Life and Work of Sigmund Freud, Vol. 1: The Formative Years and the Great Discoveries, 1856–1900*. New York: Basic Books, 1953.

Kamperidis, Lambros. "Introduction." In *The Murderess*. Edited by Nikos D. Triandaphyllopoulos. Translated by Liadain Sherrard. Limmi, Evia: Denise Harvey, 2011/1903.

Kimball, Meredith M. "From 'Anna O.' to Bertha Pappenheim: Transforming Private Pain into Public Action." In *History of Psychology*, 20–43. Vol. 3 (1), 2000.

Klossowski, Pierre. *Sade, My Neighbor*. Translated by Alphonso Lingis. Evanston, IL: Northwestern University Press, 1991/1947.

Krafft-Ebing, Richard von. *Psychopathia Sexualis: The Classic Study of Deviant Sex*. Translated by Franklin S. Klaf. New York: Arcade Publishing, 2011/1886.

Krauss, Rosalind E. "Entropy." In *Formless: A User's Guide*, 73–78. Edited by Krauss, Rosalind E. and Yve-Alain Bois. New York: Zone Books, 1997.

Lacan, Jacques. "Beyond Castration Anxiety." In *Anxiety: The Seminar of Jacques Lacan, Book X*, 43–54. Edited by Jacques-Alain Miller. Translated by A. R. Price. Malden, MA: Polity Press, 2018/1962.

Laing, Ronald David. *The Divided Self: An Existential Study in Sanity and Madness.* Baltimore, MD: Penguin Books, 1970.

Leiris, Michel. *La Possession et ses aspects theatreaux chez les Ethiopiens de Gondar.* Paris: Le Sycomore, 1980/1958 (French).

Lévi-Strauss, Claude. *Tristes Tropiques.* Translated by John and Doreen Weightman. New York: Atheneum Press, 1978.

Lewis, Ioan Myrddin. "Trance, Possession, Shamanism, and Sex." In *Anthropology of Consciousness*, 20–39. Vol. 14 (1), 2003.

Loewald, Hans W. "Psychoanalysis as an Art and the Fantasy Character of the Psychoanalytic Situation." In *Papers on Psychoanalysis*, 352–371. New Haven, CT: Yale University Press, 1980.

Luhrmann, Tanya. "Trance." In *The Dictionary of Anthropology*, 471–472. Edited by Thomas Barfield. Malden, MA: Blackwell Publishers, 2001.

Maroda, Karen. "Book Review: A Dream of Undying Fame: How Freud Betrayed His Mentor and Invented Psychoanalysis, and: Sigmund Freud and the History of Anna O.: Reopening a Closed Case." In *American Imago*, 677–686. Vol. 67 (4) Winter, 2010.

McKenzie, Karen and George Murray. "Psychotherapy as Entropy Management." In *Medical Hypotheses*, 156–158. Vol. 81, 2013.

Mitchell, Stephen. *Relational Concepts in Psychoanalysis: An Integration.* Cambridge, MA: Harvard University Press, 1988.

Mitchell, Stephen. *Relationality: From Attachment to Intersubjectivity.* Hillsdale, NJ: The Analytic Press, 2000.

Modell, Arnold H. "A Narcissistic Defense against Affects and the Illusion of Self-sufficiency." In *International Journal of Psychoanalysis*, 275–282. Vol. 56, 1975.

Morin, Edgar 1989. "Approaches to Nothingness." In *Looking Back on the End of the World*, 81–95. Edited by Dietmar Kamper and Christoph Wulf. Translated by David Antal. *Semiotext(e).* Foreign Agent Series, New York: Columbia University, 1989.

Morton, Timothy. *Dark Ecology: For a Logic of Future Coexistence.* New York: Columbia University Press, 2016.

Nietzsche, Friedrich. "On the Uses and Disadvantages of History for Life." In *Untimely Meditations*, 57–123. Edited by Friedrich Nietzsche. Translated by Reginald John Hollingdale. New York: Cambridge University Press, 1992/1874.

Oesterreich, Traugott Konstantin. *Possession: Demoniacal and Other Among Primitive Races, in Antiquity, the Middle Ages, and Modern Times.* Translated by David Ibberson. New Hyde Park, NY: University Books, 1966/1921.

Ogden, Thomas 1989. "The Initial Analytic Meeting." In *The Primitive Edge of Experience*, 169–194. Edited by Thomas Ogden. Northvale, NJ: Jason Aronson, 1989.

Pappenheim, Bertha. "Letter from Bertha Pappenheim to Robert Binswanger, November 8, 1882." In *The Life and Work of Josef Breuer: Physiology and Psychoanalysis*, 304–305. Edited and translated by Albrecht Hirschmuller. New York: New York University Press, 1978a/1882.

Pappenheim, Bertha. "Poem." In *The Life and Work of Josef Breuer: Physiology and Psychoanalysis,* 308. Edited and translated by Albrecht Hirschmuller. New York: New York University Press, 1978b/1911.

Pappenheim, Bertha [pseudonym Paul Berthold]. *In the Junk Shop and Other Stories.* Translated by Renate Latimer. Riverside, CA: Ariadne Publishing, 2008/1911.

Parke, H. W. *Sibyls and Sibylinne Prophecy in Classical Antiquity.* Edited by B. C. McGing. New York: Routledge, 1988.

Pollock, George H. "Gluckel von Hamelin: Bertha Pappenheim's Idealized Ancestor." In *American Imago*, 216–227. Vol. 28 (3), 1971.

Pollock, George H. "Bertha Pappenheim: Addenda to Her Case History." In *Journal of the American Psychoanalytic Association*, 328–332. Vol. 21 (2), 1973.

Pollock, George H. "Anna O.: Insight, Hindsight, and Foresight." In *Anna O.: Fourteen Contemporary Reinterpretations*, 26–33. Edited by Max Rosenbaum and Melvin Muroff. New York: Free Press, 1984.

Proust, Marcel. *Swann's Way: In Search of Lost Time, Vol. 1.* Translated by C. K. Scott Moncrieff and Terence Kilmartin. Revised by D. J. Enright. New York: Modern Library, 2003/1913.

Rousseau, Jean-Jacques. *Confessions.* Translated by Angela Scholar. New York: Oxford University Press, 2008/1782.

Sacher-Masoch, Leopold von. "Venus in Furs." In *Masochism*, 143–272. Translated by Jean McNeil. New York: Zone Books, 1991/1870.

Safouan, Moustahpa. "The Story of Anna O.: A Revision." In *PsychCritique: The International Journal of Critical Psychology and Psychoanalysis*, 47–54. Vol. 2 (1), 1987.

Schafer, Roy. *Language and Insight.* New Haven, CT: Yale University Press, 1978.

Shorter, Edward. "What was the Matter with 'Anna O': A Definitive Diagnosis." In *Freud Under Analysis: History, Theory, Practice*, 23–34. Edited by Todd Dufresne. Northvale, NJ: Jason Aronson, 1997.

Showalter, Elaine. "Hysteria, Feminism, and Gender." In *Hysteria Beyond Freud*, 286–344. Edited by Elaine Showalter. Berkeley, CA: University of California Press, 1993.

Shur, Max. *Freud: Living and Dying.* New York: International Universities Press, 1972.

Simmel, Georg. "Metropolis and Mental Life." In *The Sociology of Georg Simmel*, 409–424. Edited and translated by Kurt H. Wolff. New York: Free Press, 1964/1903.

Smithson, Robert. "Entropy and the New Monuments." In *The Collected Writings*, 10–23. Edited by Jack Flam. Berkeley, CA: University of California Press, 1996a/1966.

Smithson, Robert. "Entropy Made Visible." In *The Collected Writings*, 301–309. Edited by Jack Flam. Berkeley, CA: University of California Press, 1996b/1973.

Sontag, Susan. "The Pornographic Imagination." In *A Susan Sontag Reader*, 205–233. Edited by Raymond James Sontag. New York: Vintage Books, 1983.

Sontag, Susan. *Against Interpretation and Other Essays.* New York: Anchor Books, 1990.

Spence, Donald. *Narrative Truth and Historical Truth: Meaning and Interpretation in Psychoanalysis.* New York: W. W. Norton & Company, 1982.

Sulloway, Frank J. *Freud: Biologist of the Mind.* Cambridge, MA: Harvard University Press, 1992.

Swenson, Carol R. "Freud's 'Anna O.': Social Work's Bertha Pappenheim." In *Clinical Social Work Journal*, 149–163. Vol. 24 (2), 1994.

Taussig, Michael. *Mimesis and Alterity: A Particular History of the Senses*. New York: Routledge, 1993.

Wier, Dennis. *Trance: From Magic to Technology*. Ann Arbor, MI: Trans Media, 1996.

Wikipedia. "Killer BOB." Retrieved from: https://en.wikipedia.org/wiki/Bob_(Twin_Peaks).

Yapko, Michael. *Trancework: An Introduction to the Practice of Clinical Hypnosis, 3rd Edition*. New York: Brunner-Routledge, 2003.

Pandemic postscript
Screened out

I first heard from a colleague that therapists were resorting to teletherapy, virtual psychotherapy, or technologically mediated psychotherapy (I still do not know what to name it). My resistance gave way to fearful acceptance. All the patients I regularly meet accepted the offer of this new form of treatment (distance therapy?). All except one. Nico left an unequivocal message on my voicemail, stating that he would not continue with me until we could meet in person. In my unthinking haste to facilitate the transition of my entire practice population onto an altered representational platform, I barely had time to register the meaning of this sole dissent. Nico's decision inadvertently reflected the social dimension of a practice that sustained itself, at least partly, through reflexive, ritual compliance and reliance. For most, the generalized discomfort with the ensuing disruption was indistinguishable from the anxiety over contracting a potentially fatal illness. Without a choice in the matter everyone gave it a go, except Nico.

Nico, too, was terrified of exposure but not to the virus. He was terrified by the screen that would now mediate our connection (WhatsApp, Zoom, FaceTime, Skype, etc.). Nico knew that the screen presented a challenge to his ability to both present himself and relate to, or even identify with, my translated representation of him. The fear in his voice when he begged off the offer to phone it in betrayed a nearly phobic avoidance. It was as though he might be found out. But why? From a distance, and without his participation, I continued to be haunted by him and his withdrawal.

Nico is a very big, morbidly obese man, born and raised in a Mediterranean country, who communicates as much with his whole body as his vocal cords. Approximately 40 years old, he works in Manhattan as a chef. He presides over a very demanding restaurant kitchen with several assistants where he is simultaneously overstressed and grateful for the daily, unrelenting challenge that drowns out the voices in his head.

From childhood, Nico wrestled with internal voices, invariably unkind and critical, that never leave him in peace. As an adult, he sought to quiet them with cocaine, alcohol, prostitutes, and generally dangerous living. Now he's sober and attends Alcoholics Anonymous meetings whose combination of slogans and social reinforcement are barely holding him together. He randomly met a colleague of mine in Riverside Park and, appealing to him for relief, procured my name. He had never been in treatment before and was desperate.

Nico anxiously entered our first session seeming as though he were about to explode. He could not sit still or stop moving. Through his heavy accent I got the impression that he was quite self-aware, or at least in the way that 12-step patients in "recovery" can seem. Paramount in his history was a father that he described as "crazy." Apparently, his father also heard voices, operated in another reality, and seemed poorly related, if even accessible, to Nico in childhood. Understandably, Nico was concerned that he was just a chip off the old block.

When Nico pressed for immediate relief from his debilitating, paranoid anxiety I suggested a medication consult which he rejected. He was, after all, in recovery from substances and deeply suspicious of any chemical solution. I decided to conduct a hypnotic session with him in which I would simply attempt (and gauge his ability) to have him relax. The experience was unusual; with his eyes closed he felt as though I was continuously moving throughout the induction, now close, then far away, which frightened him. He left a message after this session to cancel all future therapy but after a few weeks called me back, again quite desperate, asking to continue. His staff had filed complaints against him, his only child said he could not stand to be in the same room with him, and his AA cohort pitied him from a distance. What could I do for him?

Nico required a partition, a divide between the real and the imaginary that he could not construct himself. He sought a reliable screen that enabled a notion or experience of himself as distinct from the non-him, from his father, from the voices. I believe that in our sessions he was searching for that screen in my body, not in anything I said. If in session I was calm, he was calm; if I was distressed, so was he. Maybe someday I would be his trusted mirror in which cognition and recognition occur, but for now I was less seen then felt as the auxiliary parasympathetic affective system he appropriated, borrowing my somatic ability to control myself and self-regulate in his presence. My body yielded somatic cues as to how I was able to exist as an autonomous "I" amid the roaring stimulation from the past and the present, from inner and outer space.

Bertram Lewin (1973) postulated the presence of a screen as the developmental baseline for all human interaction:

> The dream screen, as I define it, is the surface onto which a dream appears to be projected. It is the blank background, present in the dream though not necessarily seen, and the visually perceived action in ordinary dream contents takes place on it or before it.

88

Lewin goes on to trace the infantile discovery of the screen as embodied in the mother's breast. This would seem to be a prelude to symbolic activity, in much the same way as a white page enables the print you are now reading.

Beyond being a prerequisite for individual symbolic activity, the screen is intrinsically related to what it means to be human. "There can never have been a moment when specularity was not at least in part constitutive of human subjectivity ... And ever since the inception of cave paintings, it has been via images that we see and are seen" (Silverman 1996, 195).

Not only is the specularity of the screen ubiquitous, but it invariably holds a double function as both revealing and partitioning. Moreover, this dual property of the screen is often associated, in the anthropological imagination, with the site of the cave (as distinct from the breast). The suggestion of a prehistoric prototype for the screen, that both reveals and partitions, predates even Plato's cave with its spectacular allegory dividing real and ideal forms.

It is in the Neolithic paintings of the Lascaux caves that Bataille (1955) locates the original point at which the screen emerges as the intermediary partition between animals and humans. Some speculation is offered as to how these paintings could have developed accidentally from the protohumans (Cro-Magnon) mimetically copying bears with whom they alternately shared the caves and who left scratches on the walls. These primitive marks developed into paintings that possibly coincided with, or supported, the development of language. Such nascent classificatory activities led to a distinction between human and animal, a highly ambivalent and tentative distinction that we can imagine, with Bataille, was experienced perhaps more as a loss than an achievement. (In the same way, analogously, that the elaboration of a dream relayed through secondary process narrative never quite recaptures the immediacy of primary process experience.)

Bataille (1992a) speaks of the cave paintings as a kind of play, much like eroticism, and the striking degree to which this play (over thousands of years) was linked to an awareness of death that further reinforced the arbitrary division of animal and human. "The image of man and/as beast exists as an irreconcilable combination of eroticism and death, identification and displacement, affirmation and negation" (Kendall 2009, 31). But, Bataille warns, the inner connection to the animal and the animal life would never be completely lost and would forever haunt humans from within: "The definition of the animal as a thing has become a basic human given. The animal has lost its status as man's fellow creature, and man, perceiving the animality in himself, regards it as a defect" (Bataille 1992b: 39). Rules – of grammar, kinship, religion, and so on – would be constructed as the bulwark against any threat of a return.

Psychologically speaking, Lacan cites the "Nom/Non" of the father as the quintessential rule that facilitates admission into the Symbolic realm. Observing this single (metaphorical) law, representing eons of cultural development in itself, is required for the child to join society and leave dreams of merger (incest) derivative of animality behind (the foundational importance of the incest taboo for the rise of human culture is famously asserted by Lévi-Strauss 1969). For the rest of our lives, nagging anxiety dreams of arriving for a test or a performance completely unprepared will linger as relics of the fear of not passing the test posed by the "Nom/Non." But what happens when the test is administered by a psychotic father?

Nico was living as an imposter. He never took the test, or he tried and failed. He faked an ability to decipher signification and, like so many psychotically paranoid individuals, was terrified of being found out and persecuted. How did he pass all these years before I met him? He was expert in mimetically matching the tenor, tone, inflexion, accent of each person he met – and of hiding/tolerating the voices in his head. Until now.

Nico's creative, albeit furtive, blend of tactility, mimesis, and "as if" served him well in the kitchen where he apprenticed and taught others, far from the observation of hungry diners waiting outside. Now, in pandemic lockdown, he sits at home, eating, sleeping, masturbating, seeking distraction in silence, defenseless against the voices that disrupt "the *continuum* that distinguishes the animal realm" (Richman 2018, 157, author's emphasis).

Nico is off our grid, screened out, unrepresentable, and invisible to those of us who made the passage, via the new Nom/Non, into the virtual cave, protected behind our screens against the contagion of inter-species communion.

New York City, April 2020

Bibliography

Bataille, Georges. *Lascaux or the Birth of Art: Prehistoric Painting.* Translated by Austryne Wainhouse. New York: Skira Publishers, 1955.

Bataille, Georges. *The Tears of Eros.* Translated by Peter Connor. San Francisco, CA: City Lights Books, 1992a.

Bataille, Georges. *Theory of Religion.* Translated by Robert Hurley. New York: Zone Books, 1992b.

Kendall, Stuart. "Introduction." In *The Cradle of Humanity: Prehistoric Art and Culture*, 9–31. Edited by Stuart Kendall. Translated by Michele Kendall and Stuart Kendall. New York: Zone Books, 2009.

Lévi-Strauss, Claude. *The Elementary Structures of Kinship.* Edited by Rodney Needham. Translated by James Bell, John von Sturmer, and Rodney Needham. Boston, MA: Beacon Press, 1969.

Lewin, Bertram. "Sleep, the Mouth, and the Dream Screen." In *Selected Writings of Bertram D. Lewin*, 87–100. Edited by Jacob A. Arlow. New York: Psychoanalytic Quarterly, Inc, 1973/1946.

Richman, Michele. "Bataille's Prehistoric Turn: The Case for Heterology." In *Theory, Culture, & Society*, 115–173. Vol. 35 (4–5), 2018.

Silverman, Kaja. *The Threshold of the Visible World.* New York: Routledge, 1996.

Index

Note: *Italic* page numbers refer to figures.